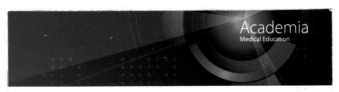

Academia
Medical Education

Provided as part of the Academia
Medical Education program.

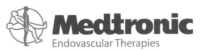

Medtronic
Endovascular Therapies

Advanced Hybrid and Endovascular Aortic Surgery

Advanced Hybrid and Endovascular Aortic Surgery

A Case-based Approach

by

Robert O. Mitchell, MD

Director of Aortic Surgery
Central Baptist Hospital
Lexington, KY, USA

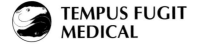

TEMPUS FUGIT
MEDICAL

NOTICE

Knowledge and best practice in the field of medicine and surgery are constantly changing. This
text consists of cases performed by the author for illustrative purposes only. No drugs, dosages,
techniques, or products are promoted by the author, publisher, or device manufacturer in this
text. Ultimately all treatment choices must be determined by and be the responsibility of the
treating physician/surgeon based upon their knowledge and experience and tailored to the needs
of their fully informed patient and in accordance with accepted practice standards and the
indications for usage (I.F.U.) as indicated by the Food and Drug Administration guidelines. To the
fullest extent of the law neither the publisher or author of this text assume any liability for
injury/damage to person or property arising out of or related to any use of the material contained
in this book.

Publisher

Library of Congress Cataloguing-in-Publication Data
Advanced hybrid and endovascular aortic surgery / by Robert O. Mitchell.

ISBN: 978-0-615-55772-4
Library of Congress Control Number: 2011942120
A catalogue record for this book is available from the Library of Congress.

Set in 9.5/13pt Minion by BAKER COMMUNICATIONS
Printed in the United States by API, Inc., Cincinnati, Ohio USA
Case Binding by Bindtech, Inc., Nashville, Tennessee USA
2012

Contents

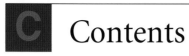

Contents

Contents

Preface

My initial goal in writing this textbook was to capture the current state of the art in endovascular and aortic surgery. This proved much more difficult than I originally thought as by the time a chapter or section was written, new information emerged and new technology became available. Indeed some of the procedures and terminology used to describe a particular surgery would differ in just a few months for the description of a very similar problem in another patient.

My secondary goal was to produce a text by a single author as opposed to an edited version with many authors. Most textbooks today are written by multiple authors who are recognized for their expertise, research, or high-volume in a specific area of surgery. They are often at large academic centers scattered throughout the United States and abroad. Certainly, edited books may be the best source of reference information on a particular topic. However, I wanted to give a glimpse into how one surgeon, in one town, in one community hospital must manage patients with a number of different pathologies. Each case scenario described in this book represents a patient in my practice whose surgery I performed. Yet, any favorable outcomes are not mine alone as on each surgery I was assisted by one of my outstanding partners. The patients also benefited from a talented team of consulting physicians and a dedicated nursing staff.

Finally, I realize that books themselves are a dying breed. Currently, much of the surgical information is disseminated through web-based publications. That is a trend that will not stop. However, there is something about putting a pen to paper that helps one clarify their thoughts and the computer monitor will never speak to me like the ink on a page. Also, many web-based articles are not subject to the peer review process. To that end, I have invited a number of physicians who are recognized experts in cardiac and vascular surgery to provide a critical commentary at the end of each chapter. No commentaries were excluded and no commentaries were edited. It is only by allowing others to objectively and critically evaluate our work that we can achieve the best clinical outcomes for our patients.

Robert O. Mitchell, MD

Foreword

There is never a time when surgery is not in need of vision. In fact, sometimes we as a discipline require the most vision when we think we are already seeing the farthest. At every turning point, there have always been a few trailblazers as imaginative as Joseph Lister and as remarkable as the general anesthetic relief of pain. A most memorable quote that I heard at a young stage in my life came from one of the most creative of plastic and reconstructive surgeons when he said, "Life is never easy on the frontier; you just must be sure you are right and then go full speed ahead." Thus said D. Ralph Millard, MD, F.A.C.S. That was his attribution to the wisdom and creativity that marked his own career and certainly marks this book by Robert Mitchell.

In surveying the evolution of genuine advances in surgery, it seems to me that inevitably the problem patient becomes the mother of invention. One of the many unusual aspects of this book is that it is a unique example carried out by someone with ingenuity, technical expertise and no lack of imagination who is a leader in practice. Interestingly in the field of surgery, only vascular surgery was quick to embrace interventional techniques and assume a leadership position in such endeavors. Few cardiac surgeons chose to attempt to add either minimally invasive or interventional radiologic approaches to these endeavors. But this book is a perfect example of how one can accomplish such.

My introduction to Robert O. Mitchell actually came through a telephone call from the most senior respected surgeon in this Commonwealth, Branham Baughman, MD, F.A.C.S., from Frankfort, Kentucky. He pointed out that a most talented young man from our state capital had been admitted to Centre College and that it was my duty to be sure that he became an enrollee at our medical school. Needless to say, Robert was a superior undergraduate and an exceptional resident, who repeatedly turned away my efforts to seduce him into a career in academic general surgery and, instead, pursued further training in cardiac surgery. The best outcome of this decision was that he ultimately returned to Kentucky within a few miles of his hometown and has continued to make imaginative contributions not just to Kentucky but also to the world of surgery.

Curiously cardiothoracic surgeons in very small numbers chose to marry the techniques of endovascular surgery and open cardiac surgery to include valve replacement. Had you asked me a decade ago who would be the person to undertake this kind of endeavor and make it successful, Robert Mitchell would have been on my very short list! This book is its own testimony; I commend it to readers for the innate imagination and creativity involved with the treatment of each of these patients and the perfection of each of these operations.

Hiram C. Polk Jr., MD

Foreword

The evolution of vascular surgery over the past two decades represents a metamorphosis from classical operative procedures – often referred to the "cut and sew" era – to endovascular therapy concentrating on the less invasive approaches, particularly those where percutaneous routes can be applied. Historically in the endovascular arena, the "hot tip" laser became a short-lived fad with only minimal contribution to improving arterial flow. On the other hand, it raised interest in working from within the lumen of the vessel and when the first arterial stents became available to solve the dissection, thrombosis and rupture problems resulting from balloon angioplasty, endovascular was forever alive.

Not surprisingly, vascular surgeons did not immediately accept this revolutionary paradigm shift in patient management. Most lacked catheter – based skills and were excluded from operative imaging facilities; thus turf wars ensued. Now the pendulum has swung back to a new, practical and exciting period of hybrid endovascular surgery. Dr. Mitchell in this text created upon a case-based approach expresses the epitome of this current vascular evolution. The previous limitations of open procedures and those performed percutaneously are to a great extent reduced or eliminated with these hybrid approaches. In reality, this represents an amalgamation to create better outcomes even for the most advanced and complex vascular pathologies.

As I was sitting preparing this forward a new textbook appeared on my desk. I am one of the three editors with over 75 contributing authors. I could not help note the difference between Dr. Mitchell's contributions and this new textbook. His real-life, front-line, daily personal experience and approach are contrasted in the more classical multi-author contributions usually representing the reviewed work from university and institutional programs. Not to in any way be critical of the latter, but to emphasize for the practicing vascular surgeon and for those physicians who will ultimately be responsible for directing their patients for vascular interventions, this work documents the very practical experience of a single surgeon working in a community hospital and the decision making and technical expertise he applies in his every day practice.

For me, who has been very much involved in the endovascular evolution, it is refreshing to witness the creativity of this author and commend him on both his clinical work and this educational contribution.

Edward B. Diethrich, MD

F Foreword

Traversing parallel careers, Rob Mitchell and I crossed paths early in the arena of aortic endografting. Several times, I have visited Rob at his program in Lexington and he has spent time with me here in Knoxville, at the University of Tennessee Medical Center. Frequently, we have talked shop, reviewed strategies for difficult cases and shared technical tips and tricks. Working shoulder to shoulder with Rob, I have learned first hand what this monograph clearly demonstrates – that is the energy, creativity and drive characterizing Rob Mitchell's approach for treating patients with aortic conditions.

Over the past decade, we have experienced spectacular changes in the field of aortic surgery. This evolution has pressed for hybrid skill sets in surgeons advancing the field. Proficient in cardiothoracic surgery, peripheral vascular surgery and endovascular surgery, Rob Mitchell has elite expertise to pioneer aortic endovascular advances.

This book is a case-based compendium of demanding aortic conditions and masterful solutions. The cases are elegantly illustrated and each serves as a foundation for a scholarly review of the specific disease state. It will be an outstanding resource to endovascular surgeons, and all clinicians treating patients with aortic disease.

Scott L. Stevens, MD

Commentators

Joseph S. Coselli, MD
Cullen Professor of Surgery and Chief of Cardiothoracic Surgery
Michael E. DeBakey Department of Surgery
Baylor College of Medicine
Chief of Adult Cardiac Surgery
Texas Heart Institute
Houston, Texas

Edward B. Diethrich, MD
Medical Director Arizona Heart Foundation
Phoenix, Arizona

Dennis R. Gable, MD
Vice Chairman Department of Surgery
Chief of Vascular Surgery
Baylor Regional Medical Center
Plano, Texas

Baron L. Hamman, MD
Chairman Department of Cardiothoracic Surgery
Baylor University Medical Center
Dallas, Texas

Kenneth L. Mattox, MD
Professor and Vice Chairman
Michael E. DeBakey Department of Surgery
Baylor College of Medicine
Chief of Surgery and Chief of Staff
Ben Taub General Hospital
Houston, Texas

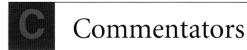

Commentators

Hiram C. Polk Jr., MD
Ben A. Reid, Sr. Professor of Surgery, Emeritus
Department of Surgery
University of Louisville, School of Medicine
Louisville, Kentucky

Hazim J. Safi, MD
Professor and Chairman
Cardiothoracic and Vascular Surgery
The University of Texas Medical School at Houston
Houston, Texas

Scott L. Stevens, MD
Professor of Surgery
Director of Endovascular Surgery
University of Tennessee Medical Center
Knoxville, Tennessee

Abbreviations

AAA	Abdominal aortic aneurysm
rAAA	Ruptured abdominal aortic aneurysm
ACF	Aortocaval fistula
ACTA2	Gene encoding smooth muscle alpha actin
ADAM	Aneurysm detection and management (trial)
ARSA	Aberrant right subclavian artery
AUI	Aortouniiliac
BF	Bifurcated
CIAA	Common iliac artery aneurysm
COL3A1	Gene encoding type III procollagen
cm	Centimeter
CRP	C-reactive protein
CT	Computerized tomography
CTA	Computerized tomographic angiogram
C-TAG	Conformable - thoracic aortic endograft
DREAM	Dutch randomized endovascular management (trial)
ECM	Extracellular matrix
EDS	Ehlers-Danlos syndrome
EEG	Electroencephalographic
ELG	Endoluminal graft
EVAR	Endovascular aortic aneurysm repair
EVOR	Endovascular aortic occlusive repair
FBN1	Fibrillin-1
FDA	Food and Drug Administration
Fr	French
ICU	Intensive care unit
IVC	Inferior vena cava
IVUS	Intravascular ultrasound
LDS	Loeys-Dietz syndrome
LSCA	Left subclavian artery
MEP	Motor evoked potential
MFS	Marfan syndrome

Abbreviations

mm	Millimeter
MMPs	Matrix metalloproteinases
MRA	Magnetic resonance angiogram
MRI	Magnetic resonance imaging
MYH11	Gene encoding smooth muscle myosin heavy chain
OVER	Veteran's Affairs open versus endovascular repair (trial)
PAA	Para-anastomotic aneurysm
PAI-1	Plasminogen activator inhibitor - 1
PTFE	Polytetrafluoroethylene
SVC	Superior vena cava
TAA	Thoracic aortic aneurysm
TAAA	Thoracoabdominal aortic aneurysm
TAAD	Thoracic acute aortic dissection
TAG	Thoracic aortic graft
TAVI	Transcatheter aortic valve implantation
TEVAR	Thoracic endovascular aortic aneurysm repair
TGFBR1	Transforming growth factor - B receptor 1 gene
TGFBR2	Transforming growth factor - B receptor 2 gene
UKSAT	United Kingdom small aneurysm trial

Manufacturer Information

AFX™ Stentgraft	Endologixs, Inc., Irvine, CA
Amplatz occluder™	AGA Medical Corp., Plymouth, MN
AneuRx™	Medtronic Corp., Santa Rosa, CA
C-TAG™	W. L. Gore and Associates, Flagstaff, AZ
Captivia™	Medtronic Corp., Santa Rosa, CA
CardioMEMS™	CardioMEMS, Inc., Atlanta, GA
CoilTrac™	Medtronic Corp., Santa Rosa, CA
CoreValve™	Medtronic Corp., Santa Rosa, CA
Dacron™	DuPont, Kingston, NC
E-vita™	JOTEC, Hechingen, Germany
Endurant™	Medtronic Corp., Santa Rosa, CA
Excluder™	W. L. Gore and Associates, Flagstaff, AZ
Gianturco Z Stent™	Cook Medical Inc., Bloomington, IN
iCAST™	Atrium Medical Corp., Hudson, NH
Lunderquist™	Cook Medical Inc., Bloomington, IN
Multilayer Flow Modulator	Cardiatis, Isnes, Belgium
Palmaz™	Johnson and Johnson Intervention, Warrendale, NJ
Powerlink™	Endologixs, Inc, Irvine, CA
Proform-TX2™	Cook Medical Inc., Bloomington, IN
Propaten™	W. L. Gore and Associates, Flagstaff, AZ
Siena™	Vascutek, Inc., Ann Arbor, MI.
Smart stent™	Johnson and Johnson Interventions, Warrendale, NJ
Solopath™	Onset Medical, Irvine, CA
Somanetics™	Covidien, Mansfield, MA
TAG™	W. L. Gore and Associates, Flagstaff, AZ
Talent™	Medtronic Corp., Santa Rosa, CA
Tearaway™ Sheath	Galt Medical Corp., Garland, TX
Valiant™	Medtronic Corp., Santa Rosa, CA
Viabahn™	W. L. Gore and Associates, Flagstaff, AZ
Wallstent™	Boston Scientific Corp., Natick, MA
Xcelerant™	Medtronic Corp., Santa Rosa, CA
Zenith™	Cook Medical Inc., Bloomington, IN

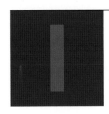

SECTION I
Abdominal Aortic Aneurysms

CHAPTER 1

Abdominal Aortic Aneurysms: Natural History, Etiology, Genetics, Medical Therapy

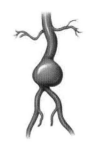

The life so short, the skill so long to learn.
— Hippocrates

The last several decades have seen significant advancements in the understanding of abdominal aortic aneurysms (AAAs) and thoracic aortic aneurysms (TAAs). Epidemiologic studies have identified familial clustering among patients with AAAs as well as other risk factors contributing to the development and progression of aneurysmal diseases. Genetic research has furthered our understanding of the generalized connective tissue disorders such as Marfan syndrome and Type IV Ehlers-Danlos syndrome; both long implicated with aneurysm formation. Biochemical studies are continuing to elucidate the role of specific matrix metalloproteinases (MMPs) and circulating inflammatory mediators in the pathogenesis of aneurysms. This chapter is to provide a brief overview of the current understanding of abdominal aortic aneurysms.

AORTIC RUPTURE AND COST

Ruptured abdominal aortic aneurysms (AAAs) are the 10th leading cause of death among men older than 55 years.[1] Most studies demonstrate a mortality rate of less than 5% for elective surgical repair of AAAs. Operative rates for open surgical repairs of ruptured AAAs vary between 40 to 50%.[2-4] Given that nearly 50% of patients with aortic ruptures die before reaching the hospital and that 30% die at the hospital without undergoing surgery,[5] the overall mortality of a patient with a ruptured AAA is 90%.

Clearly the ability to identify the significant AAA and proceed with elective repair is far better for the patient. In addition to the emotional cost paid by the patient and their family, the treatment of ruptured AAAs is an economic burden on the health care system and society. A study in the United Kingdom concluded that $50 million and 2,000 lives could be saved annually if aneurysms were treated prior to rupture.[6] If extrapolated to the more populous United States, the overall cost of aortic rupture would be far greater as 8,500 in-hospital death were attributed to ruptured AAAs in 1991.[7] A more recent study concluded that emergency repairs of ruptured AAAs result in a financial loss to the hospital of $24,655 per patient.[8] In addition to the significantly greater chance of patient death, the financial cost of emergency aortic repairs is five fold the cost of elective aortic repair.[9]

ANEURYSM DEFINITION

Precisely defining what constitutes an aortic aneurysm has been somewhat controversial. Some authors define an infrarenal aorta with a transverse diameter of greater than or equal to 3 cm as aneurysmal. Other authors define an aneurysm as a focal dilation at least 50% larger than the expected normal diameter of a given artery.[10, 11] It is important to understand that the above description only applied to attempts to define when the abdominal aorta becomes aneurysmal. These definitions do not directly imply a significant risk of rupture or the need to surgically repair a 3 cm aneurysm.

ABDOMINAL AORTIC ANEURYSM INCIDENCE

Abdominal aortic aneurysms primarily affect men over 50 years of age. Aneurysms are 2 to 6 times more common in men than woman and 3 times more common in white men than African American men.[7, 12, 13] In men, AAAs tend to occur at 50 years of age and reach a peak incidence at 80 years of age. In women, the onset of AAAs is delayed by 10 years compared with men. Women begin to develop AAAs at 60 years of age and that incidence increases steadily throughout life.[14-16] In an ultrasound screening study of United States Veterans, new AAAs were detected in 2.6% of patients 4 years after an initial normal aortic ultrasound. This yields an incidence of 6.5 per 1,000 patient-years.[17]

ABDOMINAL AORTIC ANEURYSM INCIDENCE OF RUPTURE

The natural history of AAAs is one of growth and expansion. Large prospective studies have documented AAA expansion rates at 2.6-3.3 mm per year.[18, 19] Other studies have demonstrated a growth rate of 0.3-0.5 mm per year.[20-22] Larger aneurysms tend to grow faster than smaller aneurysms.

The pioneering work of Dr. Szilagyi and others in the late 1960s confirmed the increasing risk of aneurysm rupture with increasing size. These studies provided the basis for the recommendations of early surgical repair.[23, 24] It should be noted that the aortic measurements in these early studies were based on physical examination and abdominal roentgenograms. Both of these modalities are known to overestimate AAA size by nearly 1 cm. Therefore, reported risks of rupture in these early studies for a 6 cm AAA may actually indicate the risk of rupture of a 5 cm AAA.

Potential Rupture Rates for an AAA of a Given Size (26)

AAA Diameter (cm)	Rupture Risk (% / yr.)
< 4	0
4-5	0.5-5
5-6	3-15
6-7	10-20
7-8	20-40
> 8	30-50

Table 1-1 Potential rupture rates for an AAA of a given size.[26]

Modern studies have shown an incidence of AAA rupture at 76 per 100,000 person-years for men and 11 per 100,000 person-years for women in a population base 50 years of age or older. The median age of rupture was 76 years in men and 81 years in women. The median size of AAAs at time of rupture was 8 cm; however it is important to note that **4.5% of all AAA ruptures were in aneurysms smaller than 5 cm.**[25] Table 1-1 indicates relative rupture risk as percent/year for a given aortic diameter. This table was published as guidelines for treatment strategies by the Society of Vascular Surgery in 2003.[26] Table 1-1 is only a guideline for relative risk of rupture in a large population base; it does not imply a specific risk to an individual patient or a size at which surgery is indicated.

UNITED KINGDOM SMALL ANEURYSM TRIAL (UKSAT)

A recent and often-quoted study of AAA risk of rupture is the UKSAT. Their trial demonstrates the annual risk of rupture was 1.5% for AAAs with a diameter of 4.0 to 4.9 cm, and 6.5% for AAAs 5.0 to 5.9%.[18,27,28] The authors concluded no survival advantage for early surgery versus careful surveillance for aneurysms less than 5.5 cm. However, there are some nuances to this trial that merit attention. First, the real risk of rupture of small AAAs may be underestimated as a number of patients in the surveillance group underwent repair of the AAAs either for rapid expansion or the development of symptoms. Ultimately, greater than 60% of patients initially randomized to the surveillance group crossed into the surgery group after a median of only 2.9 years of surveillance. Secondly, only 17% of the trial participants were women and they had a 4.5 fold higher risk of rupture than men. Other studies have indicated that the average diameter of a ruptured AAA is 0.5 cm smaller in women than in men.[29] Third, mortality for the elective surgery group in the UKSAT was 5.8%. A mortality of 5.8% for elective AAA repairs is higher than the mortality in most major United States medical centers. This adds further confusion in recommending which size AAAs should be repaired. Patients in the surveillance group that crossed over into the surgical group consisted of more ruptures and emergency repairs and had an operative mortality of 7.2%.

ANEURYSM DETECTION AND MANAGEMENT STUDY (ADAM)

The ADAM study was conducted with 1,163 United States Veterans with known AAAs with a diameter of 4.0 to 5.4 cm.[19,32] Patients were randomized to early surgery versus ultrasound surveillance at 6 month intervals. Patients unlikely to be compliant with surveillance were excluded. After a mean follow-up of 4.9 years, no survival benefit was noted among patients randomized to early surgery versus surveillance. Operative mortality in the surgical group was 2.7%. However, just as in the UKSAT, 60% of surveillance patients crossed over into the surgical group during the study period. Twenty-seven percent of patients with initial AAA

diameter of 4.0 to 4.4 in the surveillance group ultimately underwent surgery. The ADAM trial supported the finding of the UKSAT that elective surgery for AAA less than 5.5 cm offers no survival benefit over careful surveillance for most patients. However, the majority of patients carefully followed did ultimately require surgery. The ADAM trial did have only 1% female patients and females are known to rupture their aneurysms at a smaller size. Also, as mentioned, patients likely to be noncompliant were excluded from the ADAM trial.

Another study among United States Veterans indicated that 30% of patients were not compliant with surveillance ultrasounds despite multiple appointment reminders. Ten percent of these noncompliant patients experienced aneurysm rupture.[30] The above studies provide guidelines for the surgical management of the asymptomatic patient with an AAA. However, it is important to remember that all symptomatic aneurysms usually require repair regardless of size and that a patient is best served by an experienced surgeon carefully considering a patients gender, family history, aneurysm size and shape, risk factors, and the likelihood of patient compliance.

RISK FACTORS FOR AAA DEVELOPMENT

A number of risk factors have been implicated in the development of AAAs. These factors include: cigarette smoking, advancing age, male gender, obesity and hypercholesterolemia. Of these factors, hypercholesterolemia may be more associative and less causative than once thought. Cigarette smoking by both numbers of cigarettes smoked and years of smoking contributes the highest relative risk of aneurysm development. The relative risk of having an AAA of greater than 4 cm is 5-fold higher in smokers than in non smokers.

Table 1-2 lists the odds-ratio of detecting an unknown AAA of greater than or equal to 4 cm by independent risk factors.[17] Cigarette smoking is more likely associated with the development of an AAA than it is with either coronary or cerebral

**Independent Risk Factors for
Detecting 4 cm or Larger AAA
During Ultrasound Screening** (17)

Risk Factor	* Odds Ratio
Smoking History	5.1
Coronary Artery Disease	1.5
COPD	1.2

* Odds ratio indicates relative risk in comparison to patients without risk factor.

Table 1-2 Independent risk factors for detecting 4 cm or larger AAA during ultrasound screening.[17]

vascular disease. A history of "ever-smoking" and developing an AAA in men is 2.5 times more likely than "ever-smoking" and developing coronary artery disease and 3.5 times more likely than developing cerebrovascular disease.[17, 31-34] Other pooled studies of over 3 million patients have confirmed the relative risk impact of cigarette smoking with the development of AAAs.[35] Although male gender imparts an increased risk for aneurysm formation as compared with female gender, the relative risk of rupture for a given size aneurysm is greater in females. A number of studies have generated conflicting conclusions as to whether hypertension independently is a risk factor for aneurysm formation; however, hypertension has been more clearly associated with the rupture of established AAAs. [17, 36-39]

FAMILIAL CLUSTERING AND GENETICS

Familial clustering of patients with AAAs is well documented and underlying genetic defects are probably causative. It is well established that patients with Type IV Ehlers-Danlos syndrome have mutations with exon deletions in the gene coding

for Type III procollagen. The resulting weakened collagen in the aortic wall leads to early aneurysm formation and aortic rupture.[40, 41] Patients with Marfan syndrome have mutations in the FBN1 gene which codes Fibrillin-1. Fibrillin-1 is a glycoprotein and a major component of the microfibrils that form elastin in the aortic wall.

Aside from the above mentioned syndromes with their specific genetic defects, there are also patterns of AAA clustering among families. Familial association is so prevalent and consistent among gender that an underlying genetic defect is almost certainly involved. However, the complex interplay between environmental risk factors and genetics make elucidating an exact etiology technically and statistically challenging. In one of the most thorough studies, aortic ultrasound examinations were conducted on 87 asymptomatic brothers and sisters of 32 patients who had undergone aortic aneurysm surgery. On initial ultrasound, 29% of the brothers and 6% of the sisters all had an aortic aneurysm.[42] A supporting study demonstrated that if asymptomatic siblings of a patient with an AAA are screened by ultrasound, aneurysms can be detected in 25% of male and 7% of female siblings.[43] Of patients undergoing surgery for an AAA, ultrasound screening has demonstrated 25% of their first-degree relatives over the age of 50 years have an AAA as compared to only 2-3% of age-matched control patients. Overall, first-degree relatives of a patient with an AAAs will have a 18-fold increased risk aneurysm development in their lifetime as compared with the general population. Additionally, patients identified as part of a familial AAA cohort have their aneurysm development an average of 7 years sooner than patients with non-familial sporadic aneurysms.[44-51]

An interesting 9-year prospective study of 542 consecutive patients undergoing surgery for an AAA was reported by the surgeons at Massachusetts General Hospital. First-degree relatives with AAA were detected in 15% of the families of these surgical patients. This is very similar to findings reported by other researchers. However, of the patients that experienced aneurysm rupture, there was a female first-degree relative in their pedigree 63% of the time. (Significance P < 0.05). Thus, the presence of female members of a familial cluster may be a marker for the potential for early aneurysm rupture.[47] Again this would apply only to females as part of a familial cluster, not to females with sporadic non-familial aneurysms.

MATRIX METALLOPROTEINASES (MMPs)

Matrix metalloproteinases (MMPs) are Zn^{2+}-dependent endopeptidases of the superfamily metzincins. They have been called collagenases or gelatinases in the early literature because they degrade collagen. Twenty-five MMPs have been identified in humans and the most studied in regards to AAA formation and rupture are MMP-2 and MMP-9. These MMPs can essentially degrade all of the extracellular matrix substances of the aortic wall. They have been implicated in the pathogenesis of TAAs and AAAs for more than a decade.[52, 53] Plasma levels of MMP-9 are known to increase in patients with AAAs. Levels of MMP-9 are also increased in aneurysmal aortic tissues as compared to tissue from normal sized aortas. Patients with AAAs less than 4 cm in diameter have lower levels of MMP-9 than do patients with AAAs of 5 to 6.9 cms.[54-57] Patients that have had aneurysm repair by either open surgery or endovascular surgery consistently have reduced levels of circulating MMP-9. There is evidence that if a patient develops a significant endoleak after endo-AAA repair, the levels of plasma MMP-9 will increase.[58, 59] The implications of obtaining a biomarker for aneurysm and/or endoleak development are significant. If simple blood tests can detect an aneurysm or endoleak it will greatly reduce the need for expensive computerized tomography and the associated radiation exposure.

INFLAMMATORY AND AUTOIMMUNE FACTORS

Inflammation has long been associated with aortic aneurysm disease. The aortic wall matrix is constantly remodeling and releasing degradation products in the normal healing process. The elastin degradation products stimulate mononuclear chemotaxis and phagocytosis.

Inflammatory cell signaling and chemotaxis are mediated by cytokines such as tumor necrosis factor and the interferons. The very complex interplay between cellular immunity, proinflammatory signals, and proteinases is not fully understood. Proinflammatory compounds in cigarette smoke lead to increased production of oxidizing radicals such as superoxides (O_2^-) and peroxides (H_2O_2). The oxidized radicals inhibit the enzyme plasminogen activator inhibitor-1 (PAI-1). PAI-1 functions to inhibit and limit the deleterious effects of MMPs.[60, 61]

Although it might be expected that general biomarkers for inflammation such as C-reactive protein (CRP) would be elevated in patients with AAAs, the levels of CRP in enlarging asymptomatic AAAs has been inconsistent. In patients with symptomatic or ruptured AAAs, increased levels of CRP are more consistent.[62, 63]

Some chronic autoimmune diseases have been associated with the development of aneurysms. Aneurysms are frequently identified in patients with Kawasaki disease, Wegener's granulomatosis, and Takayasu disease.

BIOCHEMICAL AND HEMODYNAMIC FACTORS

The aorta is not a rigid tube, but an elastic structure susceptible to the forces of the cardiac cycle. Each of the segments along the length of the aorta are exposed to differing degrees of force and wall stress. When compared to the suprarenal aorta, the infrarenal segment is exposed to increased wall shear stress, increased peripheral resistance, and reduced flow when a person is in a seated position. This may explain the 5-fold increase in incidence of abdominal aortic aneurysms as compared with thoracic aortic aneurysms.

Although not well understood, it has been recognized that sedentary lifestyles predispose to arterial wall degeneration as an independent risk factor.[64] It has also been recognized that spinal cord injury with lower extremity paralysis may predispose to aneurysm formation.[65] Similarly, high above knee amputations have been associated with an increased risk of aneurysm formation.[66] Each of these scenarios result in decreased distal blood flow and increased peripheral resistance to blood flow; factors implicated in aneurysm formation. Currently a large scale trial is underway to evaluate the benefit of supervised lower extremity exercise in reducing the progression of small AAAs.[67]

MEDICAL TREATMENT OF AAAs

The most certain and definitive therapy for significant AAAs remains surgical intervention. For many years the medical management of aortic aneurysms consisted primarily of blood pressure control and finger-crossing. However, as our understanding of the pathophysiology of aneurysms has evolved, other treatment modalities are showing promise. The potential implications of even a moderately successful medical therapy are significant. Since most aneurysms grow slowly at only 2 to 3 mm per year and since most patients are 60 to 70 years of age when their aneurysm is diagnosed, a therapy that would slow aneurysm growth rate by only 50% might prevent the need for surgery in the patient's lifetime.

TOBACCO CESSATION

First and foremost, patients must discontinue smoking. Several reports demonstrate an association between continued cigarette smoking and more rapid aneurysm expansion.[68-70] Smoking cessation is the single most important aspect of medical therapy.

BETA-BLOCKERS

Beta-blockers have been postulated to decrease AAA expansion by stabilizing the matrix proteins of the aortic wall and reducing the biomechanical stress forces on the aorta.[71] Two large trials failed to demonstrate a reduction in aneurysm expansion with the use of propranolol.[72, 73] However, both trials were compromised by a high noncompliance rate of the participants.

STATINS

Two uncontrolled observational trials concluded that aneurysm expansion rates were less in patients taking statins compared with patients not taking statins.[74, 75] Both trials were nonrandomized and subject to bias. At this time it is still unclear whether it is beneficial to prescribe statins based on the diagnosis of AAA alone.

TETRACYCLINES

Two small prospective randomized trials using doxycycline at a dose of 150-200 mg/day resulted in a decreased rate of aneurysm expansion.[76, 77] Although doxycycline has antibacterial activity against Chlamydia Pneumoniae, an organism often found in the wall of AAAs, it is felt that doxycyclines ability to inhibit MMPs is its primary mode of action. Consensus guidelines for the use of doxycycline do no exist, however some physicians are using this drug for patients unable to undergo surgery. Questions remain regarding appropriate dosage and duration of treatment. Also, side effects of nausea and light sensitivity are not insignificant.

EXERCISE

As mentioned earlier, a sedentary lifestyle, spinal cord injury, and above knee amputations have been linked to aneurysm formation. Trials are ongoing with supervised lower extremity exercise as a means to slow AAA expansion. It seems intuitive that patients with small aneurysms who can ambulate should be advised to be in a regular walking routine.

COMMENTARY

(Dennis R. Gable, Plano, TX) This chapter provides an excellent broad overview that will be useful for both the layman reading this text as well as the practitioner in active practice. The chapter provides information stemming from the origin of aneurismal disease and what current theories are for the cause and development of aortic aneurysms. It covers options for current for medical and surgical therapy as well as some more recent data for indications of surgical treatment. It is an excellent beginning to a book on aortic disease.

REFERENCES

1. Prevention CDC: Leading Causes of Death, United States, 2000-2005. www.cdc.gov. 2008.

2. Hallin A, Berggvist D, Holmberg L. Literature Review of Surgical Management of Abdominal Aortic Aneurysm. *European Journal of Vascular and Endovascular Surgery.* 2001; 22: 197-204.

3. Heller JA, Weinberg A, Arons R, et al. Two Decades of Abdominal Aortic Aneurysm Repair: Have We Made Any Progress? *Journal of Vascular Surgery.* 2000; 32: 1091-1100.

4. Bowne MM, Sutton AJO, Bell PR, Sayers RD. A Meta-Analysis of 50 Years of Ruptured Abdominal Aortic Aneurysm Repair. *British Journal of Surgery.* 2002; 89: 714-730.

5. Bengtsson H, Bergqvist D. Ruptured Abdominal Aortic Aneurysm: A Population-Based Study. *Journal of Vascular Surgery.* 1993; 18: 74-80.

6. Pasch AR, Ricotta JO, May AG, et al. Abdominal Aortic Aneurysm: The Case For Elective Resection. *Circulation.* 1984; 70 (3 part 2): I 1-14.

7. Gillum RI. Epidemiology of Aortic Aneurysm in the United States. *Journal of Clinical Epidemiology.* 1995; 48: 1289-1298.

8. Breckwoldt WL, Mackey WC, O'Donnell Jr TF. The Economic Implications of High-Risk Abdominal Aortic Aneurysms. *Journal of Vascular Surgery.* 1991; 13: 798-803.

9. Cota AM, Omer AA, Jaipersad AS, et al. Elective Versus Ruptured Abdominal Aortic Aneurysm Repair: A 1-Year Cost-Effectiveness Analysis. *Annals of Vascular Surgery.* 2005; 19 (6): 858-861.

10. Johnston KW, Rutherford RB, Tilton MD, et al. Suggested Standards for Reporting on Arterial Aneurysms. Subcommittee on Reporting Standards for Arterial Aneurysms, Ad hock Committee on Reporting Standards, Society for Vascular Surgery and North American Chapter, International Society for Cardiovascular Surgery. *Journals of Vascular Surgery.* 1991; 13: 452-458.

11. Pearce WH, Slaughter MS, LeMaire S, et al. Aortic Diameter as a Function of Age, Gender, and Body Surface Area. *Journal of Surgery.* 1993; 114: 691-697.

12. Blanchard JF. Epidemiology of Abdominal Aortic Aneurysms. *Epidemiology Review.* 1999; 21: 207-221.

13. LeMorte WW, Scott JE, Memzoidan JO. Racial Difference in the Incidence of Femoral Bypass and Abdominal Aortic Aneurysmectomy in Massachusetts: Relationship to Cardiovascular Risk Factors. *Journal of Vascular Surgery.* 1995; 21: 422-431.

14. Bengtsson H, Bergquist D, Sternby NH. Increasing Prevalence of Abdominal Aortic Aneurysms. A Necropsy Study. *European Journal of Surgery.* 1992; 158: 19-23.

15. Melton 3rd LJ, Bickerstall LK, Hollier LH, et al. Changing Incidence of Abdominal Aortic Aneurysms: A Population-Based Study. *American Journal of Epidemiology.* 1984; 120: 379-386.

16. McFarlane MJ. The Epidemiologic Necropsy for Abdominal Aortic Aneurysm. *Journal of the American Medical Association.* 1991; 205: 2085-2088.

17. Lederle FA, Johnson GR, Wilson SE, et al. Yield of Repeated Screening for Abdominal Aortic Aneurysm After a 4-Year Interval. Aneurysm Detection and Management Veterans Affairs Cooperative Study Investigations. *Archive of Internal Medicine.* 2000; 260: 1117-1121.

18. The United Kingdom Small Aneurysm Trial Participants. Long-Term Outcomes of Immediate Repair Compared with Surveillance of Small Abdominal Aortic Aneurysms. *New England Journal of Medicine.* May 9, 2001; 346 (19): 1445-1452.

19. Lederle FA, Johnson GR, Wilson SE, et al. Immediate Repair Compared with Surveillance of Small Abdominal Aortic Aneurysms. *New England Journal of Medicine.* May 9, 2002; 346 (19): 1437-1444.

20. Englund R, Hudson P, Hanel K, et al. Expansion Rates of Small Abdominal Aortic Aneurysms. *Australian and New Zealand Journal of Surgery.* 1998; 68 (1): 21-24.

21. Hirose Y, Hamada S, Takamiya M, et al. Predicting the Growth of Aortic Aneurysms: A Comparison of Linear Versus Exponential Models. *Angiology.* 1995; 46 (5): 413-419.

22. Bengtsson H, Ekberg O, Aspelin P, et al. Ultrasound Screening of the Abdominal Aorta in Patients with Intermittent Claudication. *European Journal of Vascular Surgery.* 1989; 3 (6): 497-502.

23. Szilagyi DE, Smith RI, DeRusso FJ, et al. Contribution of Abdominal Aortic Aneurysmectomy to Prolongation of Life. *Annals of Surgery.* 1966; 164: 678-699.

24. Foster JH, Bolasny BL, Gobbel Jr WG, et al. Comparative Study of Elective Resection and Expectant Treatment of Abdominal Aortic Aneurysm. *Sura Gynecol Obstet.* 1969; 129: 1-9.

25. Choksy SA, Wilmink AB, Quick CR. Ruptured Abdominal Aortic Aneurysm in the Huntington District: A 10-Year Experience. *Annals of the Royal College of Surgeons of England.* 1999; 81: 27-31.

26. Brewster DC, Cronenwett JL, Hallett JEWY, et al. *Guidelines for the Treatment of Abdominal Aortic Aneurysms.* Report of a Subcommittee of the Joint Council of the American Associated for Vascular Surgery.

27. Brown LC, Powell JP. Risk Factors for Aneurysm Rupture in Patients Kept Under Surveillance. UK Small Aneurysms Trial Participants. *Annals of Surgery.* 1999; 230: 289-296.

28. The UK Small Aneurysm Trial Participants. Mortality Results for Randomized Controlled Trial of Early Surgery or Ultrasonographic Surveillance for Small Abdominal Aortic Aneurysms. *Lacet.* 1998; 352: 1649-1655.

29. Fillinger MF, Racasin J, Baker RK, et al. Anatomic Characteristics of Ruptured Abdominal Aortic Aneurysm on Conventional CT Scans: Implications for Rupture Risk. *Journal of Vascular Surgery.* 2004; 39: 1243-1252.

30. Valentine RJ, Decaprio JD, Castilo JM, et al. Watchful Waiting in Cases of Small Abdominal Aortic Aneurysms – Appropriate for All Patients? *Journal of Vascular Surgery.* 2000; 32: 441-448.

31. Blanchard JI, Aermenian HK, Friesen PP. Risk Factors for Abdominal Aortic Aneurysms – Appropriate for All Patients?" *American Journal of Epidemiology.* 2000; 151: 575.

32. Lederle FA, Johnson GR, Wilson SE, et al. Relationship of Age, Gender, Race, and Body Size to Infrarenal Aortic Diameter. The Aneurysm Detection and Management (ADAM) Veterans Affairs Cooperative Study Investigators. *Journal of Vascular Surgery.* 1997; 26: 595.

33. Singh K, Bonaa KH, Jacobson BK, et al. Prevalence of and Risk Factors for Abdominal Aortic Aneurysms in a Population-Based Study: The Troms Study. *American Journal of Epidemiology.* 2001; 154: 236.

34. Mofidi R, Goldie VJ, Kelman J, et al. Influence of Sex on Expansion Rate of Abdominal Aortic Aneurysms. *British Journal of Surgery.* 2007; 94: 310.

35. Lederle FA, Nelson OB, Joseph AM. Smokers' Relative Risk for Aortic Aneurysm Compared with Other Smoking-Related Diseases: A Systematic Review. *Journal of Vascular Surgery.* 2003; 38: 329-334.

36. Vardulaki KA, Walker NM, Day NE, et al. Quantifying the Risks of Hypertension, Age, Sex, and Smoking in Patients with Abdominal Aortic Aneurysm. *British Journal of Surgery.* 2000; 87: 195-200.

37. Alcorn HG, Wolfson Jr SK, Sutton-Tyrrell K, et al. Rick Factors for Abdominal Aortic Aneurysms in Older Adults Enrolled in The Cardiovascular Health Study. *Arterioscler Thromb Vasc Biol.* 1996; 16: 693-970.

38. Smith FC, Grimshaw GM, Paterson IS, et al. Ultrasonographic Screening for Abdominal Aortic Aneurysm in an Urban Community. *British Journal of Surgery.* 1993; 80: 1406-1409.

39. Pleumeekers HJ, Hoes AW, Vander Does E, et al. Aneurysms of the Abdominal Aorta in Older Patients. The Rotterdam Study. *American Journal of Epidemiology.* 1995; 142: 1291.

40. McKusick VA. *The Ehlers-Danlos Syndrome/ Heritulde Disorders of Connective Tissue.* 4th ed. St. Louis, MO: C.V. Mosby Co; 1972, 292-371.

41. Vissing H, D'Alessio, Lee B, et al. Multi-Exon Deletion in the Procollagen III Gene is Association with Elhers-Danlos Syndrome Type IV. *Journal of Biological Chemistry.* 1991; 266: 5244-5248.

42. Bengtsson H, Norrgard O, Angquist O, et al. Ultrasonographic Screening of the Abdominal Aorta Among Siblings of Patients with Abdominal Aortic Aneurysm. *British Journal of Surgery.* 1989; 76: 589-591.

43. Webster MW, Ferrell RE, St. Jean PL, et al. Ultrasound Screening of First-Degree Relatives of Patients with an Abdominal Aortic Aneurysm. *Journal of Vascular Surgery.* 1991; 13: 9-13.

44. Salo JA, Soisalon-Soinnen S, Bondestam S, et al. Familial Occurrence of Abdominal Aortic Aneurysm. *Annals of International Medicine.* 1999; 130: 637-642.

45. Baird PA, Sadovnick AD, Yee IM, et al. Sibling Risks of Abdominal Aortic Aneurysm. *Lancet.* 1995; 346: 601-604.

46. Cronenwett JL, Likosky DS, Russell MT, et al. A Regional Registry for Quality Assurance and Improvement: The Vascular Study Group of Northern New England (VSGNNE). *Journal of Vascular Surgery.* 2007; 46: 1093-1101.

47. Darlin 3rd RC, Brewster DC, Darling RC, et al. Are Familial Abdominal Aortic Aneurysms Different? *Journal of Vascular Surgery.* 1989; 10: 39-35.

48. Johansen K, Koepsell T. Familial Tendency for Abdominal Aortic Aneurysms. *Journal of the American Medical Association.* 1986; 256: 1934-1936.

49. Frydman G, Walker PJ, Summers K, et al. The Value of Screening in Siblings of Patients with Abdominal Aortic Aneurysms. *European Journal of Vascular and Endovascular Surgery.* 2003; 26: 396-400.

50. Verloes A, Sakalihasan N, Koulischer L, et al. Aneurysms of the Abdominal Aorta: Familial and Genetic Aspects in Three Hundred and Thirteen Pedigress. *Journal of Vascular Surgery.* 1995; 21: 646-655.

51. Kuivaniemi H, Trump G, Prockop DJ. Genetic Causes of Aortic Aneurysms. Unlearning at Best Part of What the Textbooks Say. *Journal of Clinical Investigation.* 1991; 88: 1441-1444.

52. Lee M-H and Murphy G. Matrix Metalloproteinases at a Glance. *Journal of Cell Science.* 2004; 117: 4015-4016.

53. Longo GM, Wanfen X, Greiner TC, et al. Matrix Metalloproteinases 2 and 9 Work in Concert to Produce Aortic Aneurysms. *Journal of Clinical Investigation.* 2002; 110: 625.

54. Watanabe T, Sato A, Sawai T, et al. The Elevated Level of Circulating Matrix Metalloproteinase-9 in Patients with Abdominal Aortic Aneurysms Decreased to Levels Equal to Those of Healthy Controls After an Aortic Repair. *Annals of Vascular Surgery.* 2006; 20: 317-321.

55. McMillan WD, Pearce WHY. Increase Plasma Levels of Metalloproteinase 9 Are Associated with Older Aortic Aneurysm. *Journals of Vascular Surgery.* 1999; 122-127.

56. Wilson WRW, Anderstorm M, Schwalbe EC, et al. Matrix Metalloproteinase 8 and 9 are Increased at the Site of Abdominal Aortic Aneurysm Rupture. *Circulation.* 2006; 113: 434-438.

57. McMillan WD, Tamarina NA, Cipollone BS, et al. Size Matters: The Relationship Between MMP-9 Expression and Aortic Diameter. *Circulation.* 1997; 96: 2228.

58. Sangiorgi G, D'Averio R, Mauriello A, et al. Plasma Levels of Metalooproteinases-3 and -9 as Markers of Successful Abdominal Aortic Aneurysm Exclusion After Endovascular Graft Treatment. *Circulation.* 2001; 104 (12 suppl 1): 1288-1295.

59. Lorelli DR, Jean-Claude JM, Fox CJ, et al. Response of Plasma Matrix Metalloproteinase-9 to Conventional Abdominal Aortic Aneurysm Repair or Endovascular Exclusion: Implication for Endoleak. *Journal of Vascular Surgery.* 2002; 35: 916.

60. Miller Jr FJ, Sharp WJ, Fang X, et al. Oxidative Stress in Human Abdominal Aortic Aneurysms: A Potential Mediator Aneurysmal Remodeling. *Arterioscler Thromb Vasc Biol.* 2002; 22: 560.

61. Middleton RK, Lloyd GM, Bowne MM, et al. The Pro-Inflammatory and Chemotactic Cytokine Microenvironment of the Abdominal Aortic Aneurysm Wall: A Protein Array Study. *Journal of Vascular Surgery.* 2008; 45: 574.

62. Vainas T, Lubbers T, Stassen F, et al. Serum C-Reactive Protein Level in Associated with Abdominal Aortic Aneurysm Size and May Be Produced by Aneurysmal Tissue. *Circulation.* 2003; 107: 1103-1105.

63. Domanovitis H, Schillinger M, Mullner M, et al. Acute Phase Reactants in Patients with Abdominal Aortic Aneurysms. *Atherosclerosis.* 2002; 163: 297-302.

64. Gimbrone Jr MA, Topper JN, Nagel T, et al. Endothelial Dysfunction, Hemodynamic Forces, and Atherogenesis. *Annals of the New York Academy of Sciences.* 2000; 902: 230.

65. Yeung JT, Kim HJ, Abbruzzese TA, et al. Aortoiliac Hemodynamic and Morphologic Adaption to Chronic Spinal Cord Injury. *Journal of Vascular Surgery.* 2006; 44: 1254.

66. Vollmar JI, Paes E, Friesch A, et al. Aortic Aneurysms as a Late Sequelae of Above Knew Amputation. *Lancet.* 1989; 2: 834.

67. Dalman RL, Tedesco MM, Myers J, et al. AAA Disease: Mechanisms, Stratification, and Treatment. *Annals of the New York Academy of Sciences.* 2006; 1085: 92.

68. Lindholt JS, Heegaard NH, Vammen S, et al. Smoking, But Not Lipids, Lipoprotein (a) and Antibodies Against Oxidated LDL, is Correlated to the Expansion of Abdominal Aortic Aneurysms. *European Journal of Vascular and Endovascular Surgery.* Jan. 2001; 21 (1): 51-56.

69. MacSweeney ST, Ellis M, Worrell PC, et al. Smoking and Growth Rate of Small Abdominal Aortic Aneurysms. *Lancet.* Sept. 3, 1994; 344 (8923): 651-652.

70. Powell JT, Worrell P, MacSweeney ST, et al. Smoking as a Risk Factor for Abdominal Aortic Aneurysm. *Annals of the New York Academy of Sciences.* Nov. 18, 1996; 800: 246-248.

71. Boucek RJ, GunJa-Smith Z, Noble NL, et al. Modulation by Propranolol of the Lysyl Cross-Links in Aortic Elastin and Collagen of the Aneurysm – Prone Turkey. *Journal of Biochemical Pharmacology.* Jan. 15, 1983; 32 (2): 275-280.

72. Lindholt JS, Henneberg EW, Juul S, et al. Impaired Results of a Randomized Double Blinded Clinical Trial of Propanolol Versus Placebo on the Expansion Rate of Small Abdominal Aortic Aneurysms *International Angiology.* March 1999; 18 (1): 52-57.

73. Propranolol Aneurysm Trial Investigators. Propranolol for Small Abdominal Aortic Aneurysms: Results of a Randomized Trial. *Journal of Vascular Surgery.* Jan 2002; 35 (1): 72-79.

74. Sukhija R, Aronow WS, Sandhu R, et al. Mortality and Size of Abdominal Aortic Aneurysm at Long-Term Follow-Up of Patients not Treated Surgically and Treated With and Without Statins. *American College of Cardiology.* Jan. 15, 2006; 97 (20): 279-280.

75. Schouten O, van Laanem JH, Boersma E, et al. Statins Are Associated With A Reduced Abdominal Aortic Aneurysm Growth. *European Journal of Vascular and Endovascular Surgery.* July 2006; 32 (1): 21-26.

76. Mosorin M, Juronem J, Biancari F, et al. Use of Doxycycline to Decrease the Growth Rate of Abdominal Aortic Aneurysms: A Randomized, Double-Blind, Placebo-Controlled Pilot Study. *Journal of Vascular Surgery.* 2001; 34: 606-610.

77. Baxter, BT, Pearce WH, Waltke E, et al. Prolonged Administration of Doxycycline in Patients with Small Asymptomatic Abdominal Aortic Aneurysms: Report of a Prospective (Phase I) Multicenter Study. *Journal of Vascular Surgery.* 2002; 36: 1-12.

CHAPTER 2

Endovascular Repair of Abdominal Aortic Aneurysms

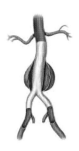

Since the first aneurysm resection and repair by Dubost in 1951, laparotomy with "open" repair has been the most widely accepted technique for abdominal aortic aneurysm surgery.[1] The reported operative mortality rates for open AAA repair range from 4% - 12%. Whereas single-centers may report mortality rates as low as 3%, large population-based studies report a mortality of 8% or higher.[2] A review of 360,000 open AAA repairs

from the hospital discharge data base demonstrate a mortality of 5.6%.[3] Clearly, the real-world statistics differ somewhat from the reports at specialized centers. In nearly all recent reports, endovascular aortic aneurysm repair (EVAR) has a significantly lower operative morality than open AAA repair.

The landmark paper by Juan Parodi detailing a series of patients treated by EVAR was published in 1991.[4] Table 2-1 lists important events in the chronology of EVAR development.[5] In 1999, the AneuRx device (Medtronic Corp, Minneapolis, MN) was the first endovascular modular system approved by the FDA to treat AAAs in the United States. Between the years 2000 and 2005, there was a 600% increase in the number of endovascular aneurysm procedures performed in United States hospitals.[9]

CHRONOLOGY OF EVAR DEVELOPMENT

1951	Open Aortic Aneurysm Repair by Dubost [1]
1969	Experimental Stent for Arterial Stenosis [6]
1990	Balloon-expandable stent-graft [7]
1990	Balloon-expandable aorto-aortic stent-graft [4]
1991	Bifurcated aortobiiliac stent-graft [8]
1996	European approval AneuRx bifurcated stent-graft
1997	European approval Excluder bifurcated stent-graft
1998	European approval Talent bifurcated stent-graft
1999	European approval Zenith bifurcated stent-graft
2002	U.S.A. approval AneuRx bifurcated stent-graft
2003	U.S.A. approval Zenith bifurcated stent-graft
2004	U.S.A. approval Powerlink bifurcated stent-graft
2010	U.S.A. approval Endurant bifurcated stent-graft

Table 2-1 Chronology of EVAR development

RANDOMIZED TRIALS OF OPEN SURGERY VS. EVAR

The EVAR-1 Trial

The EVAR-1 Trial was initiated in Great Britain in 1999. This randomized trial was designed to provide Level-1 evidence for comparing "open" versus "EVAR" aneurysm repair. The EVAR-1 Trial enrolled 1,082 patients with AAAs greater than 5.5 cm and that were candidates for either open surgery or EVAR. The 30-day mortality for patients in the EVAR group was significantly lower than for patients in the open group (1.7% vs. 4.7%, P=0.016).[10] However, four years after randomization, the "all-cause" mortality was similar in both groups at approximately 28%. The EVAR group had a higher post-procedure re-intervention rate than the open group (20% vs. 6%). Late aneurysm related deaths in the EVAR group was 4% vs. the open group of 7%.

The DREAM Trial

The Dutch Randomized Endovascular Aneurysm Management (DREAM) Trial was initiated in 1999 and also designed to yield Level-1 evidence for comparing open and EVAR repairs. The DREAM Trial contained 345 patients with AAAs greater than 5.5 cm, randomized to either EVAR or open surgery.[11, 12] The 30-day mortality results were nearly identical to the EVAR-1 Trial. Perioperative mortality was markedly less with EVAR vs. open surgery (1.2% vs. 4.6%). However, with the small number of patients, this failed to reach statistical significance. Also, as with the EVAR-1 Trial, the DREAM Trial demonstrated that the early operative mortality benefits of EVAR are lost as "all-cause" mortality at two years post procedure was 20% in both groups. Although not statistically significant, the late aneurysm related death rate with EVAR vs. open surgery was 2.1% vs. 5.7%.

The OVER Trial

The Veterans Affairs Open Versus Endovascular Repair (OVER) Trial was initiated at 41 medical centers in 2002. The trial is ongoing, but an interim report with a mean follow-up of 1.8 years was published, in 2009.[13] The trial enrolled 881 patients randomized to EVAR (n=444) or open (n=437) AAA repair. Thirty-day operative mortality was lower for the EVAR group versus the open group (0.5% vs. 3%, p=0.004). There were no major differences in the groups with regard to frequency of secondary interventions. The perioperative mortality rate, as well as the secondary intervention rate, for the EVAR group was lower than that seen in the European trials (EVAR-1 and DREAM). This could be accounted for by the inclusion of patients in the OVER Trial with aneurysms smaller than 5.5 cm, or from some other factors yet to be determined.

RANDOMIZED TRIALS FOR EVAR VS. MEDICAL THERAPY

The EVAR-II Trial

The EVAR-II Trial began in 1999 and was designed to provide Level-1 evidence comparing EVAR versus medical therapy for a group of patients deemed "unfit" for open surgical aneurysm repair.[14] Although the trial was flawed by a number of circumstances such as low numbers and cross-over between groups, still some valuable information was obtained. A total of 338 patients with AAAs greater than 5.5 cm were randomized to either EVAR (n=166) or best medical therapy (n=172). Again, all patients had been deemed high-risk and "unfit" for open surgical repair by a team of physicians.

The operative mortality for the EVAR group was high at 9%. However, this was artificially high as nine patients (5.4%) assigned to the EVAR group died of aneurysm rupture while waiting to have surgery. The medical group had a 9% risk of aneurysm rupture per year. However, this 9% annual risk of rupture is artificially low as 27% of the medical therapy group crossed-over into the EVAR group because of rapid aneurysm growth or symptoms. Interestingly, the medical group that crossed-over for urgent EVAR had only a 2% operative mortality; which was lower than that of the elective EVAR group. Remember, these were patients initially deemed to be inoperable secondary to comorbid conditions.

CONCLUSIONS REGARDING EVAR TRIALS AND CONCLUSIONS IN GENERAL

Some conclusions are obvious from the aforementioned trials and are widely accepted by most surgeons. Some conclusions have less statistical significance and are more subject to individual interpretation. A general statement regarding the above studies and how they affect my approach to patients in my real world practice follows. Some of the conclusions are subject to my personal bias.

1. First, the interpretation of major randomized trials (EVAR-I, EVAR-II, and DREAM) should be done with the understanding that EVAR techniques and devices are rapidly changing. The above three trials were initiated in 1999, nearly four years before three major endovascular devices (Excluder, Zenith, and Endologix) were approved for use in the United States. The only device approved in the United States in 1999 was the AneuRx graft; which has largely been replaced by the Talent and Endurant graft. The trials with which we make our decisions are now a decade old and the devices used in those original studies are either no longer produced or have been modified to a degree that they hardly resemble their first generation ancestors.

2. Secondly, both EVAR and open surgery have a relatively low mortality when performed by experienced surgeons. For a patient whose aneurysm is only a marginal anatomic candidate for endografting, to fall back to open surgery is not surgeon failure but sound surgical judgment.

3. In the short-term, 30-day period, the operative mortality for EVAR is less than open AAA surgery.

4. In the long-term, the survival curves for EVAR and open surgery for AAAs converge.

5. The majority of patients with AAAs under close surveillance will come to surgery.

6. The belief that open endoaneurysmorrhaphy will permanently eliminate the risk of an

aortic thrombus, and access ... influence the immediate ... of EVAR. The surgeon ... estimate of the pati... the risks of a... related de... conside... co-...

...g...y as we think (EVAR-II).

9. Even with reduced intensive care unit and hospital stays, the overall cost of EVAR is greater than that for open AAA surgery.

10. The patient will invariably choose EVAR over open surgery despite knowing EVAR's increased cost, need for surveillance, and the potential for future interventions.

11. The need for secondary interventions is probably more likely following EVAR for larger aneurysms than for smaller aneurysms.

12. Although the need for secondary interventions is more common after EVAR than open surgery, the magnitude of such interventions with EVAR is much less. Obviously the percutaneous placement of an extender cuff or embolic coils is less extensive than a repeat laparotomy for bleeding or a chyle leak.

PREOPERATIVE EVALUATION FOR EVAR

As with any surgical procedure, a careful history and physical examination should be performed by the operating surgeon. The patient's age, associated co-morbidities, and overall health must be assessed. Co-morbid conditions such as diabetes, renal insufficiency, myocardial infarction, COPD, cardiac ejection fraction, previous abdominal surgeries, and recently diagnosed malignancies must be evaluated with respect to the planned surgery. Anatomic factors such as aortic neck angulation, neck length, circumferential

vessel quality all
and long-term success
must calculate a general
ent's life expectancy and weigh
eurysm repair versus aneurysm-
th without repair; all the while
ing all-cause mortality from the patient's
orbidities. Finally, the patient's willingness
and ability to be compliant with the long-term
surveillance required of EVAR must be determined.

DIAGNOSTIC STUDIES PRIOR TO EVAR

Most patients referred to the surgeon carry a diagnosis of thoracic or abdominal aneurysm of a certain size based upon either a computerized tomographic scan or an ultrasound from an outside facility. Often, the aneurysms are an incidental finding during the evaluation of another medical condition or have been found as part of a screening examination. Most of these patients will require additional imaging modalities or more-complete studies to assess their candidacy for EVAR. I find the CT scans in which the AAA was an incidental finding most commonly lack images of the iliac and femoral arteries.

COMPUTERIZED TOMOGRAPHY

Computerized tomographic angiography (CTA) is probably the single most useful test for determining the anatomic suitability for EVAR. The axial CT images combined with 3-dimensional reconstruction provide information pertaining to nearly every aspect of EVAR. The adequate CT scan for EVAR should image from the supraceliac aorta to the common femoral arteries with axial cuts at no greater than 3 mm. I prefer 2.5 mm cuts with the 3-D reconstruction to include the proximal 2 cm of the celiac, mesenteric and renal arteries. Often importance stenoses at the origin of these branch vessels may be missed without careful attention to these areas.

Neck Diameter and Thrombus

Axial CT images provide measurements for aortic neck diameter in order to make size determinations for endograft selection. Excessively large neck diameters may exclude patients from EVAR consideration. Extensive thrombus at the level of the aortic neck may interfere with endograft seal and fixation and predispose to endoleaks and graft migration/slippage.

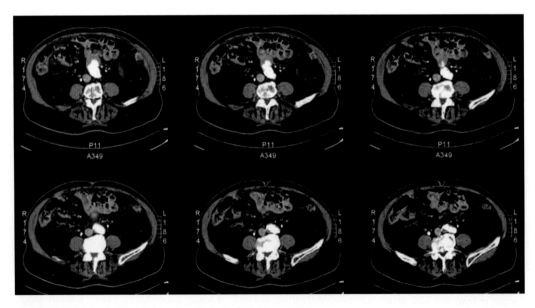

Figure 2-2 Sampling of CT axial views of an abdominal aortic aneurysm.

Access Vessel Diameter and Calcification

Axial CT measurements of iliac and femoral artery diameters are critical in determining the suitability for endograft access or if iliac conduits may be required. Computerized tomography also gives information regarding atherosclerosis and calcium burden within the access vessels. Excessive calcium in the iliac and femoral arteries suggests less distensibility of these vessels, and they are considered less-forgiving if their diameters are only marginal to accept the endograft or necessary sheaths. Axial CT images and the reconstructed 3-D images are also valuable in detecting iliac artery tortuosity and associated aneurysms of the common or internal iliac arteries.

Side-Branch Arteries

Both axial CT images and 3-D reconstructed images define the anatomic relationships of the renal and mesenteric arteries. Important areas of renal or mesenteric stenosis can be identified. Also, the take-off angles to the main body of the aorta are easily appreciated in the 3-D views. Such take-off angles are essential in positioning the side branches of fenestrated grafts.

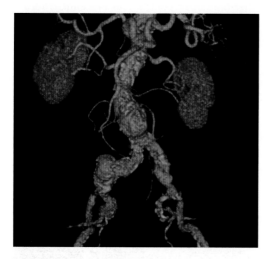

Figure 2-3 Three-dimensional reconstruction of over 170 axial views for the patient in figure 2-2. Note the angulation, right internal iliac artery aneurysm, right external iliac artery stenosis and calcium burden are easier to appreciate in a three-dimensional image.

Tortuosity

Computerized tomography is also helpful in identifying angulation and tortuosity. Although all data contained within 3-D reconstructions is present in axial images, the 3-D images can give a rapid appreciation of artery angles, tortuosity, calcium, and stenoses. Figure 2-2 is a series of CT axial views of a given abdominal aortic aneurysm. These are only a few of over 170 axial cuts that the surgeon would have to evaluate for this patient. However, figure 2-3 is one 3-D reconstruction of the same 170 axial images, which demonstrates angulation, tortuosity, and associated right internal iliac artery aneurysm, a tight right external iliac artery stenosis, and a mild to moderate calcium burden. All of this information was easily gleaned in the 3-D reconstruction seen in figure 2-3. However, to evaluate 170 images in axial cuts, some of this information may be lost.

Associated CT Findings

Computerized tomography of AAAs may yield other incidental findings. Intra-abdominal tumors, horse-shoe kidneys, and venous abnormalities may be present. Incidental findings that are deemed to be clinically significant are detected in 19% of patients undergoing CT scans prior to AAA repair.[15]

ARTERIOGRAPHY

Arteriography once played a prominent role in the preoperative planning of patients undergoing open AAA repair or EVAR. Advancements in CT angiography have greatly diminished the need for arteriography. Currently arteriography is usually performed at the time of EVAR to assess for graft length or preoperatively for embolic coiling. Figure 2-4 is an arteriogram of a fusiform abdominal aortic aneurysm.

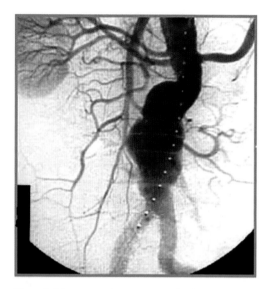

Figure 2-4 Aortogram demonstrating a fusiform abdominal aortic aneurysm. The marking catheter is used to determine curvilinear lengths.

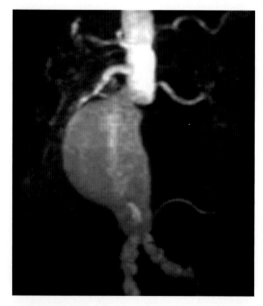

Figure 2-5 Magnetic resonance angiogram (MRA) of an abdominal aortic aneurysm.

MAGNETIC RESONANCE IMAGING

Magnetic Resonance Angiography (MRA) has an advantage over CTA in that it avoids the deleterious effects of ionizing radiation. However, MRA has a number of disadvantages and it has failed to surpass CTA as the AAA imaging modality of choice for most surgeons. Compared with CTA, MRA is more expensive, more time consuming, and not often readily available. In addition, MRA does not visualize calcium plaque well. Also, MRA techniques are more difficult to standardize due to gating techniques on different machines. Although gadolinium contrast used in MRA was once felt to be safely tolerated by patients with renal insufficiency, cases of nephrogenic sclerosing fibrosis are being reported.[16] Although CTA has become the diagnostic modality of choice for most surgeons, MRA can still provide excellent results and the concern over radiation exposure with CTA will only increase in the next few years. Figure 2-5 is an MRA representation of an AAA.

INTRAVASCULAR ULTRASOUND (IVUS)

Intravascular ultrasound (IVUS) can be used intraoperatively to locate branch ostia and to determine aortic neck diameters. However, the most significant advantage of IVUS is to determine regions of true and false lumens during repair of aortic dissections. IVUS is virtually indispensable during the endovascular repair of an aortic dissection. Figure 2-6 depicts IVUS images of an abdominal aortic aneurysm.

AORTIC NECK LENGTH

The aortic neck is considered to be the length of the aorta between the lowest renal artery and the beginning of the aneurysm. Most commercially available endografts require an aortic neck length of 15 mm. The recently approved (December, 2010) Endurant graft (Medtronic Inc., Minneapolis, MN) allows for the treatment of necks as short as 10 mm. There is evidence that aneurysms with longer necks are less likely to develop Type-I endoleaks.[17, 18]

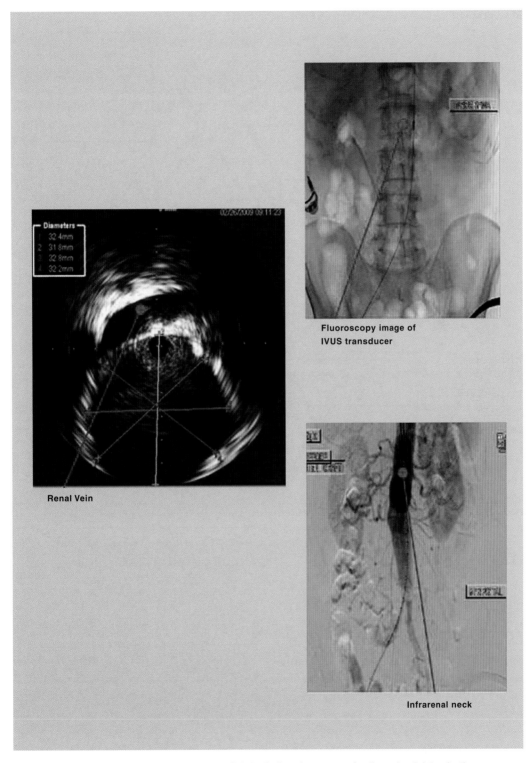

Renal Vein

Fluoroscopy image of
IVUS transducer

Infrarenal neck

Figure 2-6 Intravascular ultrasound (IVUS) images of abdominal aortic aneurysm for dimensional determinations.
Images courtesy of Volcano Corporation, San Diego, CA.

Measurements - Diameter measurements are inner wall to inner wall

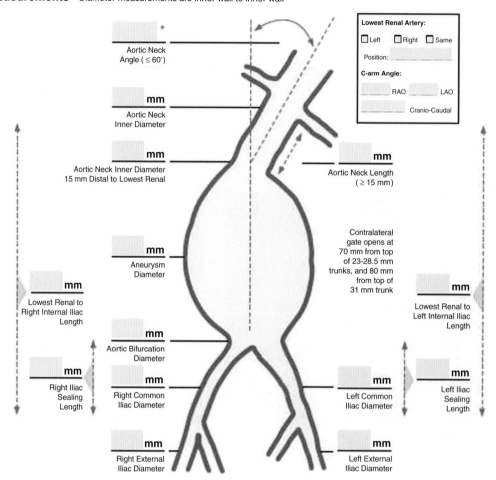

Figure 2-7 Preoperative planning worksheet for EVAR. Note the numerous dimensions which must be evaluated for successful EVAR. Illustration courtesy of W. L. Gore and Associates.

AORTIC NECK DIAMETER

Currently available endografts for AAAs can treat a maximum aortic neck diameter of 32 mm.

AORTIC NECK ANGULATION

The angle between the long axis of the aortic neck and the long axis of the main body of the aneurysm should be less than 60 degrees for favorable EVAR outcomes. Angles greater than 60 degrees predispose to endoleak and potential graft migration. Figure 2-7 is an example of a typical worksheets used to record important angles and diameters in the operative planning for EVAR.

ANEURX STENT GRAFT 1999

The AneuRx (Medtronic Inc., Santa Rosa, CA) endograft was approved by the FDA in 1999. A multicenter study enrolled 250 patients with AAAs. Sixty patients underwent open repair and 190 patients underwent EVAR. Major morbidity was 23% in the open surgical group versus 12% in the EVAR group. Ultimately over 1,190 patients were enrolled in the AneuRx arm of Phase I, II, and III of the U.S. clinical trials. The overall survival of this group was 93% and 86% at one and three years, respectively.[19, 20]

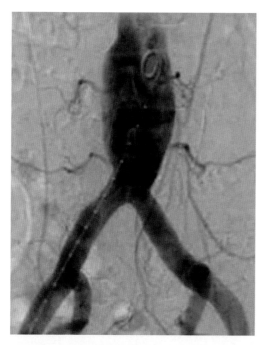

Figure 2-8 Arteriogram of abdominal aortic aneurysm prior to repair.

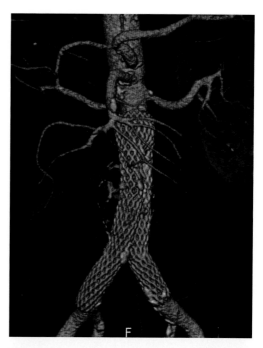

Figure 2-9 CT angiogram of abdominal aortic aneurysm of the patient in figure 2-8 seven years post repair with the Medtronic stent graft.

AneuRx Case Scenario

The patient is a 77-year-old man with a 5.3 cm AAA, hypertension, status post coronary artery bypass grafting years before. He underwent un-eventful repair with a Medtronic AneuRx device in March, 2004. The patient's preop AAA is demon-strated in figure 2-8. The endograft remains in good position without graft migration or endoleak after seven years, figure 2-9. Although the AneuRx components are still available, the latest generation Endurant graft has demonstrated excellent results and essentially replaced the AneuRx graft.

ENDURANT STENT GRAFT 2010

The Endurant stent graft system received FDA approval in December, 2010. Advantages of the En-durant design are the ability to treat AAA necks of only 10 mm in length with the suprarenal fixation system, figure 2-10. Other proposed advantages in-clude a hydrophilic low profile delivery system and M-shaped stent design that allows for greater flex-ibility in treating extreme aortic neck angulation.

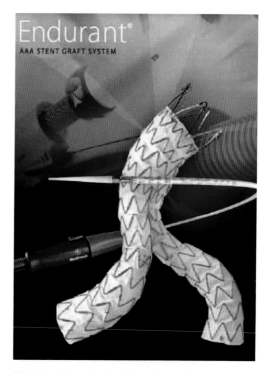

Figure 2-10 Photograph of the Medtronic Endurant graft. Photo courtesy of Medtronic Corporation.

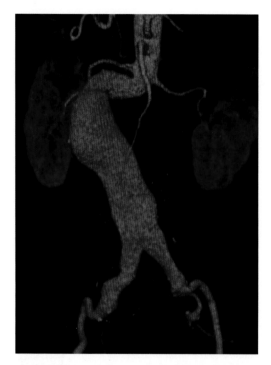

Figure 2-11 CT angiogram of tortuous infrarenal aortic aneurysm.

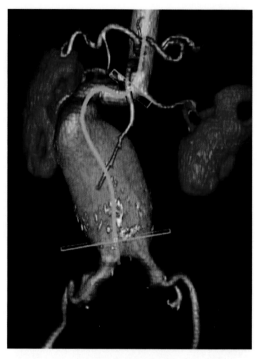

Figure 2-12 CT angiogram of same tortuous aneurysm (figure 2-11) with computerized midline demonstrating severe neck angulation (blue line).

Endurant Case Scenario

The patient is a 74-year-old man with an extremely tortuous 7.5 cm infrarenal AAA as demonstrated in figure 2-11. Bilateral femoral artery cutdowns were performed and a 0.035 inch guidewires were placed in the descending thoracic aorta under fluoroscopic visualization. Using guide catheters, these wires were exchanged for 260 cm length super-stiff 0.035 inch wires. Super-stiff Lunderquist wires were used because of the tortuosity of both the iliac arteries and the angulated aortic neck. Figure 2-12 demonstrates the angulation of this aneurysm. Embolic coils were placed in the right internal iliac artery. A 20-Fr sheath was placed via the right femoral artery and a 16-Fr sheath via the left femoral artery. The delivery system is its own self-contained device and does not require an additional sheath for insertion. However, in this case I chose to use the Endurant delivery system through a 20-Fr sheath as the

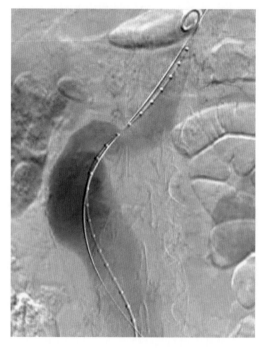

Figure 2-13 Intraoperative arteriogram prior to repair.

sheath would occlude the origin of the right internal iliac artery. The previously placed embolic coils had migrated to the ostia of the internal iliac artery and I was concerned that they might embolize into the external iliac artery. The 20-Fr sheath would keep the coils isolated until the graft extension limb secured and sealed the coils within the internal iliac artery.

The intraoperative arteriogram prior to graft placement is seen in figure 2-13. The Endurant graft, size 32 mm x 16 mm x 16 cm, was deployed without difficulty below the renal arteries. The extreme tortuosity of the aorta made cannulation of the contralateral gate difficult. Ultimately a wire was placed through the gate in antegrade fashion from above and then snared from below. The intraoperative arteriogram after AAA repair is seen in figure 2-14 and the large 20-Fr somewhat impedes runoff into the right limb of the graft. The postoperative CT angio is depicted in figure 2-15.

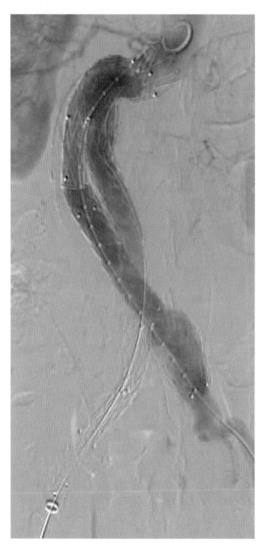

Figure 2-14 Arteriogram post repair.

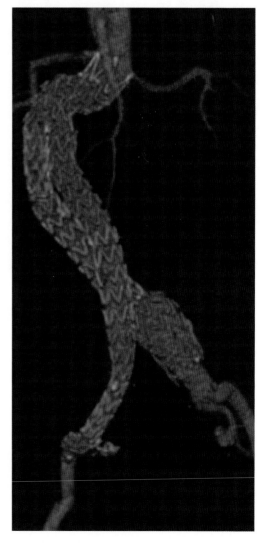

Figure 2-15 CT angiogram post aneurysm repair.

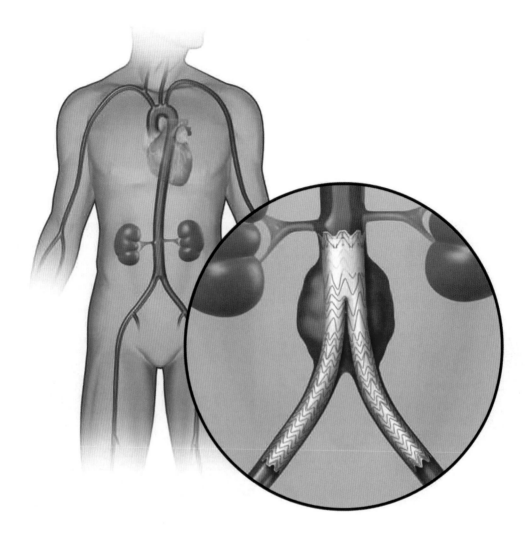

Figure 2-16 Model of Gore Excluder graft. Illustration courtesy of W. L. Gore and Associates.

EXCLUDER STENT GRAFT 2002

The Excluder is a bifurcated graft system with a self-expanding Nitinol stent and polytetrafluoroethylene (PTFE), figure 2-16. The multicenter United States Pivotal Trial compared patients treated with the Excluder endograft versus open aneurysm repair. Although no statistical difference was seen in overall survival, the endograft cohort had less blood loss, less intensive care unit stay, and faster recovery. Thus there was a significant reduction in adverse events for the endograft group compared with the open group (14% vs. 57%, p< 0.0001).[21]

Excluder Case Scenario

The patient is a 74-year-old man with a 6 cm saccular infrarenal aortic aneurysm, figure 2-17. The AAA was repaired with a Gore Excluder bifurcated stent graft, size 23 mm x 12 mm x 14 cm, main body right via an 18-Fr sheath. The contralateral limb was placed via a 12-Fr sheath in the left femoral artery. The post repair CT angio is seen in figure 2-18.

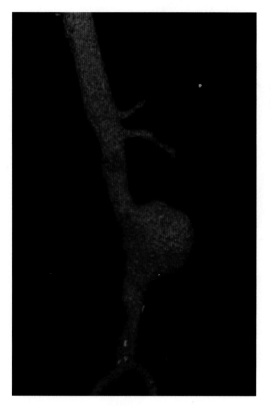

Figure 2-17 CT angiogram of 6 cm infrarenal abdominal aortic aneurysm.

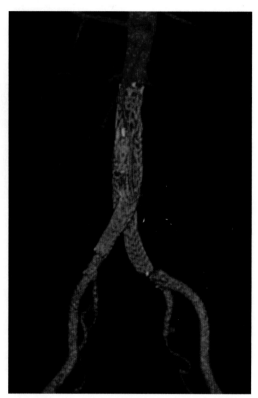

Figure 2-18 CT angiogram post AAA repair with Gore Excluder graft.

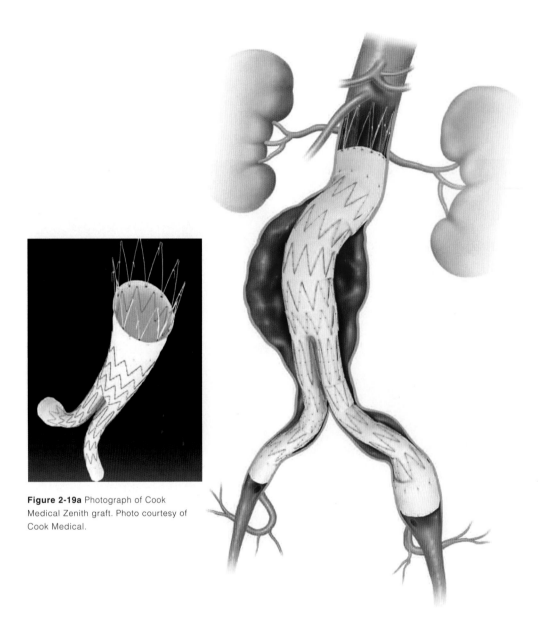

Figure 2-19a Photograph of Cook Medical Zenith graft. Photo courtesy of Cook Medical.

Figure 2-19b Photograph of Cook Medical Zenith Flex graft. Image courtesy of Cook Medical.

ZENITH STENT GRAFT 2003

The Zenith graft (Cook Medical Inc., Blooming-ton, IN) is a bifurcated endograft with stainless steel stents. It has a proximal uncovered stent extension for suprarenal attachment and fixation to the aortic wall, figure 2-19a and 19b. In a trial with over 350 patients, those with the Zenith endograft had significantly less major adverse events than the open surgical group. At 12 months post procedure, endograft migration was not detected in any patient with the Zenith endograft.[22, 23]

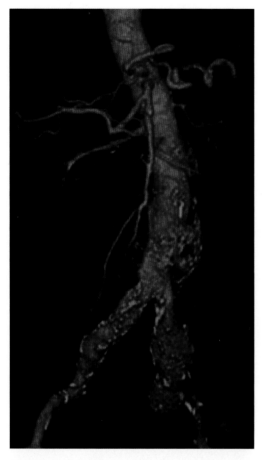

Figure 2-20 CT angiogram of infrarenal aortic aneurysm prior to repair.

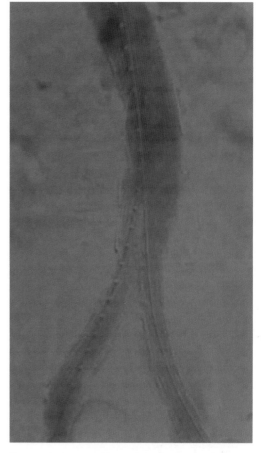

Figure 2-21 Intraoperative aortogram at time of repair of aneurysm with Zenith graft.

Zenith Case Scenario

The patient is an 84-year-old man with a 6 cm AAA and a 3 cm common iliac artery aneurysm, figure 2-20. Bilateral femoral artery cutdowns were performed and 0.035 inch guidewires were placed in the descending thoracic aorta. A 24-Fr sheath was placed via the left femoral artery and a Zenith graft (Cook Medical Inc., Bloomington, IN) size 36 mm x 95 mm length was placed. A left-sided extension limb was deployed size 12 mm x 122 mm and a right contra limb size 24 mm x 88 mm completed the repair. The intraoperative aortogram following repair is seen in figure 2-21. The patient is alive at 89 years of age with no evidence of endoleak or graft migration.

POWERLINK STENT GRAFT 2004

The Powerlink endograft received FDA approval in October, 2004. The Powerlink device is a unibody bifurcated polytetrafluoroethylene (PTFE) graft with a self-expanding internal skeleton of cobalt-chromium alloy. The Powerlink device is positioned with fixation against the aortic bifurcation and then built upward toward the renal arteries. This is in contradistinction to the other devices which are first positioned at the renal arteries and built-downward. The next generation graft from Endologix is the AFX graft system, figures 2-22, 23. Proposed advantages of the Endologix system are:

1. The unibody design eliminates potential difficulties with gate cannulation.
2. One limb of the graft can be placed percutaneously with a 9-Fr sheath.
3. Graft positioning on the aortic bifurcation mitigates against graft migration and this may help secure the graft while treating wide-necked aneurysms.[26]
4. The fabric placed external to the stent cage mitigates against cage wire fractures.

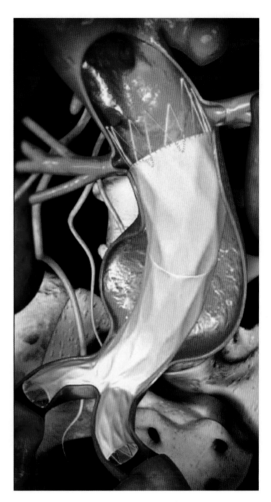

Figure 2-23 Illustration of Endologix Powerlink graft. Note graft rests distally on aortic bifurcation and also has suprarenal struts. Photograph courtesy of Endologix, Inc.

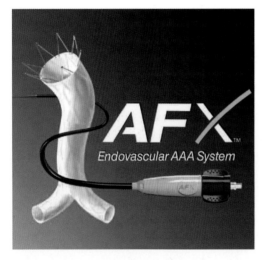

Figure 2-22 Photograph of AFX Powerlink graft. Imaging courtesy of Endologix, Inc.

The Powerlink study enrolled 258 patients between July, 2000 and March, 2003 (192 EVAR patients and 166 open repair patients). The test patients compared with controlled patients had significantly less blood loss, ICU stays, hospital stays, and myocardial infarctions. There were no ruptures, graft fabric defects, or wire fractures. An increase in native AAA diameter was noted in only 1.5% of patients at 24 months follow-up.[24, 25]

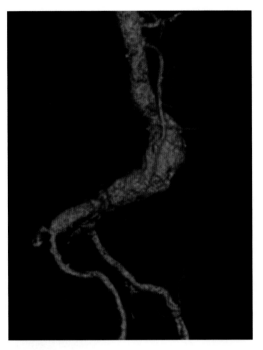

Figure 2-24 CT angiogram of tortuous aorta and iliac arteries preoperatively.

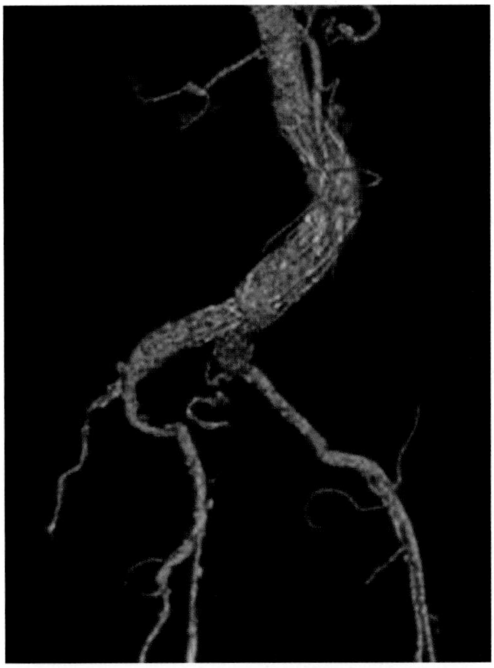

Figure 2-25 CT angiogram 4.5 years post repair with the Endologix Powerlink graft.

Powerlink Case Scenario

The patient is an 85-year-old woman with a 5.8 cm infrarenal aortic aneurysm. Note the extreme tortuosity of the aorta and iliac arteries, figure 2-24. The Powerlink device was placed via a right femoral artery cutdown. This main body was posi-tioned on the aortic bifurcation. A proximal exten-sion was built upwards and deployed to extend to the main device proximally to the level of the renal arteries. Despite the significant aortoiliac tortuosity, the graft has remained in position without endoleak or migration for the four and one half year follow-up period, figure 2-25.

COMMENTARY

(Scott L. Stevens, Knoxville, TN) In this chapter, Dr. Mitchell reviews the seismic changes we have witnessed in the field of aortic therapy over the last decade. Chronicled, are the landmark events that were pivotal to this continuum of progress. Trials providing level I data to guide physician decision algorithms are presented and key points for approaching aortic disease are outlined.

Next, the preoperative evaluation and diagnostic workup for aortic aneurysmal disease are explained. Included are the roles of ultrasound, CT scan, magnetic resonance imaging, and arteriography. Lastly, devices currently available to treat aortic pathologies are analyzed and the specific advantages for each device are characterized in clinical case scenarios.

This chapter is thorough, succinct and timely. It highlights the author's strong foundation in minimally invasive aortic therapy and will be a valuable resource for endovascular surgeons and all primary care physicians responsible for treating patients with aortic pathology.

REFERENCES

1. Dubost C, Allay M, Oeconomos N. Resection of an aneurysm of the abdominal aorta: Reestablishment of the continuity by a preserved human arterial graft, with result after five months. *AMAUROSIS FUGAX Arch Sur*g. 1952; MW; 64(3): 405-408.

2. Blankensteijn JD, Lindenburg FP, Graaf VD, et al. Influence of study design on reported mortality and morbidity rates after abdominal aortic aneurysm repair. *Br J Surg*. 1998; 85 (12): 1624-1630.

3. Cronenwett JL, Birkmeyer JD. *The Dartmouth Atlas of Vascular Healthcare*. Chicago, IL: AHA Press; 2000.

4. Parodi JC, Palmaz JC, Barone HD. Transfemoral intraluminal graft implantation for abdominal aortic aneurysm. *Ann Vasc Surg*. 1991; 5: 491-499.

5. Modified from Rutherford's Vascular Surgery, Chapter 129. Philadelphia, PA: Saunders Elsevier; 2011.

6. Dotter CT. Transluminally-placed coil-spring endoarterial tube grafts: Long-term patency in canine popliteal artery. *Invest Radiol*. 1969; 4: 329-332.

7. Laborde JC, Parodi JC, Clem MF, et al. Intraluminal bypass of abdominal aortic aneurysm: Feasibility study. *Radiology*. 1992; 184: 185-190.

8. Chuter TA, Green, RM, Ouriel K, et al. Transfemoral endovascular aortic graft placement. *J Vasc Surg*. 1993; 18: 185-195.

9. Nowygrod R, Egorova N, Greco G, et al. Trends, complications and mortality in peripheral vascular surgery. *J Vasc Surg*. 2006; Feb 43 (2): 205-216.

10. Greenhalgh RM. Brown LC, Kwong GP. EVAR trial participants. Comparison of endovascular aneurysm repair with open repair in patients with abdominal aortic aneurysm (EVAR Trial I), 30-day operative mortality results: Randomized controlled trial. *Lancet*. 2004 Sep 4-10; 464 (9437): 843-848.

11. Blankensteijn JD, deJong SE, Prinssen M, et al. Dutch Randomized Endovascular Aneurysm Management (DREAM) Trial Group. Two-year outcomes after conventional or endovascular repair of abdominal aortic aneurysm. *N. Eng J Med*. 2005 June 9; 352 (23): 2398-2405.

12. Prinssen M, Verhoeven EL, Buth J, et al. Aneurysm Management (DREAM) Trial Group. A randomized trial comparing conventional and endovascular repairs of abdominal aortic aneurysms. *N Engl J Med*. 2004 Oct 14; 351 (16): 1607-1618.

13. Lederle FA, Freischlag JA, Kyriakides TC, et al. Outcomes following endovascular versus open repair of abdominal aortic aneurysm. A randomized trial. *JAMA*. 2009; Vol 32, 14: 1535-1542.

14. EVAR Trial Participants. Endovascular aneurysm repair and outcome in patients unfit for open repair of abdominal aortic aneurysm (EVAR Trial II): Randomized controlled trial. *Lancet*. 2005; 365: 2187-2192.

15. Indes JED, Lipsitz EC, Veith FJ, et al. Incidence and significance of non-aneurysmal-related computed tomography scan findings in patients undergoing endovascular aortic aneurysm repair. *J Vasc Surg*. 2008; 48: 286-290.

16. Shabana WM, Cohan RH, Ellis JHOW, et al. Nephrogenic systemic fibrosis: A report of 29 cases. *AJR Am J Roetgenol*. 2008; 190: 736-741.

17. Greenburg RR. Abdominal aortic endografting: Fixation and sealing. *J Am Coll Surg*. 2002; 194 (1): S79-A87.

18. Stanley BB, Semmens JB, Mai Q, et al. Evaluation of patient selection guidelines of endoluminal AAA repair with the Zenith stent-graft: The Australian Experience. *J Endovasc Ther*. 2001; 8 (5): 457-464.

19. Zarins CK, White RA, Moll FL, et al. The AneuRx stent graft: Four year results and worldwide experience. 2000. *J Vasc Surg*. 2001 Feb; 33 (2 suppl): S135-145.

20. Zarins CK, White RA, Schwarten D, et al. AneuRx stent graft versus open surgical repair of abdominal aortic aneurysms: Multicenter prospective clinical trial. *J Vasc Surg*. 1999 Feb; 29 (2) 292-305; discussion 306-308.

21. Kibbe MR, Matsumura JS. Excluder investigator. The Gore Excluder U.A. Multicenter Trial: Analysis of adverse events at tow years. *Semin Vasc Surg*. 2003 June; 16 (2): 144-150.

22. Greenberg R. Zenith Investigators. The Zenith AAA endovascular graft for abdominal aortic aneurysms: Clinical update. *Semin Vasc Surg*. 2003 June; 16 (2): 151-157.

23. Greenberg R, Lawrence-Brown M, Bhandari G, et al. An update on the Zenith endovascular graft for abdominal aortic aneurysms: Initial implantation and mid-term follow-up data. *J Vasc Surg*. 2001 Feb; 33 (2 suppl): S157-164.

24. Carpenter JP. The Endograft Investigation. Multicenter trial of the Powerlink bifurcated system for endovascular aortic aneurysm repair. *J Vasc Surg*. 2002; 36: 1129-1137.

25. Carpenter JP. The Endologix Investigation. Mid-term results of the multicenter trial of the Powerlink bifurcated system for endovascular aortic aneurysm repair. *J Vasc Surg*. 2004; 40: 849-859.

26. Jordan WC Jr, Moore WM Jr, Metin JG, et al. Secure fixation following EVAR with the Powerlink XL system in wide aortic necks: Results of a prospective, multicenter trial. *J Vasc Surg*. 2009; 50: 979-986.

CHAPTER 3

Endovascular Repair of Abdominal Aortic Aneurysms with Variations of the Aortouniiliac Technique

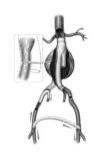

The first endovascular aneurysm repairs consisted of aorto-aortic tube grafts.[1] However, very few patients had a favorable anatomy with aortic landing-zones above and below the aneurysm to accommodate such a graft. Thus, the aortouniiliac (AUI) or aortomonoiliac repair with femoral to femoral crossover grafting emerged early in the evolution of endovascular aneurysm surgery. In the days of "homemade" endografts, the AUI devices were easy to assemble and they could be loaded and delivered with relatively small sheaths.

The use of a polytetrafluoroethylene (PTFE) graft sutured to a Palmaz stent was described and used by Frank Veith to treat a ruptured AAA as early as 1994.[2-7] The Palmaz stent could be balloon-expanded to a proximal diameter between 20 and 28 millimeters. These devices could be made in advance and would be available to treat most patients presenting with ruptured AAAs. This graft became commercially known as the Vascular Innovation (VI) Graft (Vascular Innovation, Inc., Perrysburg, OH).

Figure 3-1 illustrates the AUI repair of a ruptured AAA. The PTFE graft is sutured to a Palmaz stent and deployed proximally. The distal end of the PTFE graft is anastomosed to the femoral artery and a PTFE femoral to femoral crossover bypass is constructed. Note the occluder

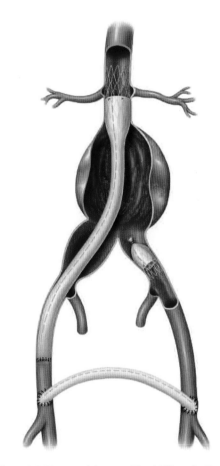

Figure 3-1 "Homemade" aortouniiliac (AUI) graft with PFTE sutured to a Palmaz stent proximally, PTFE to femoral anastomosis distally, and femoral to femoral crossover graft. Note contralateral iliac occluder.

in the contralateral common iliac artery to prevent back-filling into the aneurysm sac.

Another advantage of the AUI repair of a ruptured AAA is that is obviates the need for contralateral gate cannulation, which is required for most bifurcated graft systems. Depending upon surgeon experience and the patient anatomy, gate cannulation can be time consuming and therefore problematic in the scenario of an aneurysm rupture. The most frequent situation in which an AUI graft is used is in the case of iliac artery occlusion or severe iliac artery stenosis.

The commercially available bifurcated (BF) endografts are intuitively appealing as they more closely represent the natural anatomy. Also, the BF endografts resemble the aortobifemoral bypass with which vascular surgeons are familiar and know to have excellent patency rates. The AUI graft with femoral to femoral crossover suffers from a conceptual prejudice as it is not as anatomically appealing. Also, the femoral to femoral graft component has historically been associated with poor patency rates when performed for occlusive disease. However, the fears of femoral graft failure when combined with an AUI repair for aneurysmal disease have proved unfounded. One report demonstrates femoral to femoral patency, when associated with AUI aneurysm repair, to be 97% at 18 months.[8] Another report documents a 98% patency at 5 ½ years.[9] The Eurostar Registry contained 353 patients with AUI repairs, and reports a femoral to femoral graft patency of 97.8% at seven years.[10]

Although some reports have indicated a higher mortality among patients undergoing AUI as opposed to bifurcated endografting, those deaths were not aneurysm-related but were attributed to AUI patients being more critically ill.[11] A retrospective analysis of the Eurostar data base included 5,274 patients with a BF endograft and 353 patients with an AUI endograft. In that study 33% of the AUI patients were deemed "unfit" for open repair and only 21% of the BF patients deemed "unfit" for open repair. Although all cause mortality was

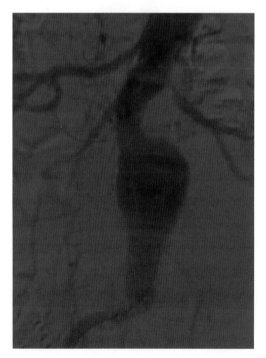

Figure 3-2 Intraoperative aortogram of 10 cm AAA with left common iliac artery occlusion.

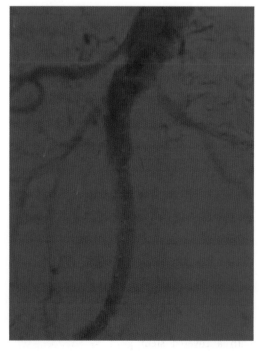

Figure 3-3 Intraoperative aortogram after AUI repair of 10 cm ruptured AAA.

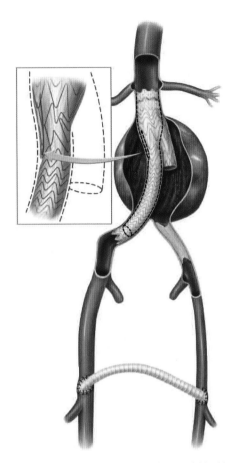

Figure 3-4 Illustration of AUI repair of 10 cm AAA with femoral to femoral graft.

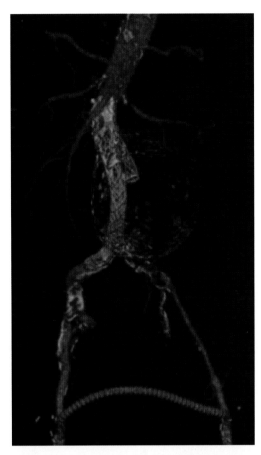

Figure 3-5 CT angiogram of AUI repair with patent femoral to femoral graft. Note calcium-outline of 10 cm aneurysm sac.

higher in the AUI group, that was attributed to the patients being older and generally more ill. However, no significant differences between the BF graft and the AUI patients were noted in respect to endoleak rate, graft migration, graft patency, and most importantly aneurysm-related death.[10]

Below are described three different case scenarios where I used variations of the AUI endograft configuration. The first case involves a straightforward AUI with femoral to femoral crossover for treatment of a ruptured 10 cm AAA. The second scenario employs the standard AUI with femoral crossover and the addition of an external iliac artery to internal iliac artery endovascular bypass with a covered stent graft to provide pelvic perfusion. The third case involves what I believe to

be one of the earliest uses of telescoping thoracic endografts in a large neck abdominal aorta to construct an AUI aneurysm repair.

CASE SCENARIO 1:
Standard AUI with Femoral Crossover

The patient is a 79-year-old man transferred from an outside hospital with back pain and a computerized tomographic scan demonstrating a 10 cm infrarenal aortic aneurysm with a contained rupture in the retroperitoneum. The femoral arteries were identified by cutdown. The left femoral artery had no pulse of significance. A pigtail catheter placed via the right femoral artery was used for an aortogram and demonstrated the

AAA and flush occlusion of the left common iliac artery at its origin, figure 3-2. An AUI repair was then performed based upon the anatomic constraints of an occluded left iliac artery. An Excluder main body endograft size 23 cm x 12 mm x 14 cm was deployed approximately 1 cm below the renal arteries. A second Excluder main body graft size 23 cm x 12 mm x 14 cm was deployed within the first graft but extending slightly above the first graft. The inner graft will occlude the orifice of the side limb of the outer graft. The side limb of the inner graft is occluded as it is compressed flat by the outer graft. Figure 3-3 is the intraoperative arteriogram after AAA exclusion using two main body grafts to create an AUI design. As now all blood flow is directed into the right femoral artery, a standard femoral to femoral crossover bypass graft was constructed with external ring supported PTFE. Figure 3-4 illustrates the completed repair. Although the side limb of the bifurcated graft would appear to be a source of endoleak, it is actually occluded from the inside by the second graft. The computerized angiographic scan demonstrates occlusion of the aneurysm, a patent femoral to femoral graft, and no evidence of retrograde endoleak, figure 3-5. The femoral graft remains patent with aneurysm exclusion over four years postoperatively.

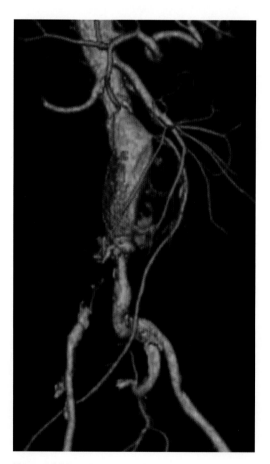

Figure 3-6 CT angiogram of AAA with right common iliac occlusion.

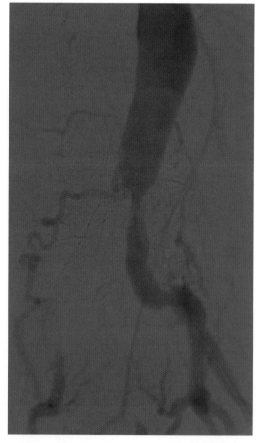

Figure 3-7 Intraoperative aortogram demonstrating AAA with right common iliac artery occlusion extending to origin of internal iliac artery.

CASE SCENARIO 2:
Standard AUI with Femoral Crossover and E to I Endobypass

The patient is a 68-year-old man with an AAA and significant bilateral thigh and buttocks claudication, right side worse than left. CT angiography shows left iliac artery stenosis, an occluded right common iliac artery and an infrarenal AAA, figure 3-6. The intraoperative arteriogram confirms the CTA findings, figure 3-7. The AUI repair was performed by first placing an Excluder main body graft into the aorta via the left femoral artery. A second Excluder main body graft was

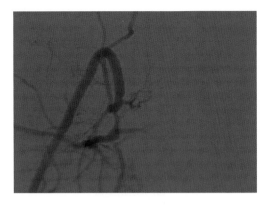

Figure 3-8 Retrograde arteriogram demonstrating flow from right external to internal iliac artery via covered endograft bypass. Note continued flow into pelvic vessels.

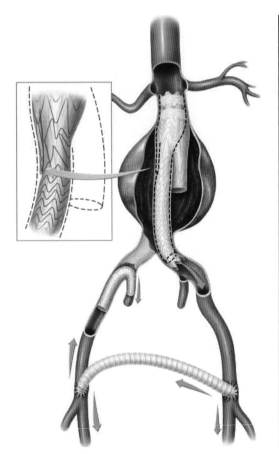

Figure 3-9 Postoperative illustration of AUI repair, left to right femoral to femoral bypass, and Viabahn graft external to internal iliac artery endobypass.

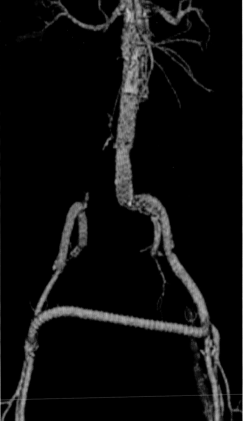

Figure 3-10 CT angiogram of AUI repair, femoral to femoral bypass and right external to internal iliac artery endobypass.

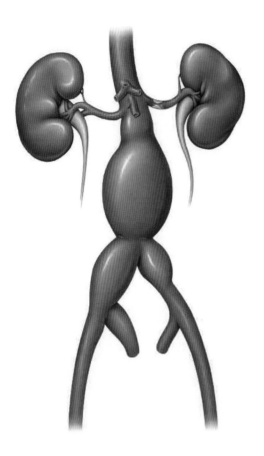

Figure 3-11 Preoperative illustration of aortic, right common iliac, and right internal iliac artery aneurysms.

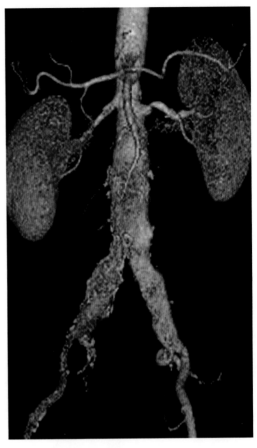

Figure 3-12 Preoperative CT angiogram demonstrating aorto-iliac aneurysm and left renal artery stenosis.

placed within the first graft and extended 0.5 cm above the first graft. As the patient's right common iliac artery was naturally occluded to the orifice of the internal iliac artery, there was no room to place embolic coils or an occluding device in the common iliac artery proper. If the coils or occluder were placed into the external iliac artery, they would prevent flow into the internal iliac artery. This problem can be solved by performing an external iliac artery to internal iliac artery (E to I) bypass with an endoluminal covered graft. Such a graft would prevent a back flow into the AAA sac should the common iliac ever recanalize. Also, the graft will provide pelvic blood flow into the internal iliac artery. The right internal iliac artery

was selectively cannulated with a soft glide wire. This wire was changed to a stiff wire and a Viabahn covered graft size 10 cm length x 7 mm diameter was deployed partially within the internal iliac artery and partially within the external iliac artery. A hand-held contrast injection via the right femoral sheath demonstrates flow from the external iliac through the graft into the internal iliac with blood supply to a rich pelvic arterial network, figure 3-8. The illustration of the completed procedure is figure 3-9. The patient maintains a patent femoral to femoral graft and is claudication free over four years postoperatively. The CT angiogram of the AUI with femoral to femoral bypass and E to I endobypass is depicted in figure 3-10.

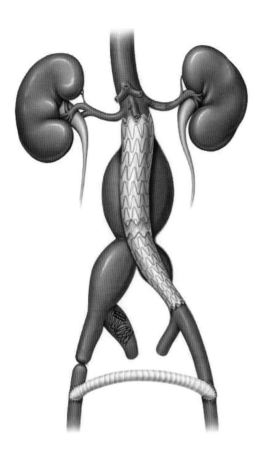

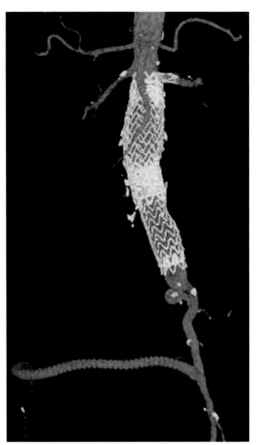

Figure 3-13 Illustration of AUI repair with telescoping thoracic endografts, femoral to femoral bypass, right internal iliac coiling, and angioplasty/stenting of left renal artery.

Figure 3-14 CT angiogram demonstrating three telescoping thoracic endografts for AUI repair, patent femoral to femoral graft, and left renal artery stent.

CASE SCENARIO 3:
AUI Utilizing Telescoping Thoracic Endografts with Femoral Crossover

The patient has an infrarenal aortic aneurysm with an enlarged neck of 30 mm diameter immediately below the renal arteries that increases to a diameter to 31 mm within a distance of approximately 0.75 cm. Additionally, there is a 3 cm right common iliac artery aneurysm and a 2.5 cm right internal iliac aneurysm, figure 3-11. The patient had a previous coronary bypass surgery, a cardiac ejection fraction of 20%, and significant pulmonary insufficiency. The patient would not likely tolerate a laparotomy and open aneurysm repair. In 2005,

I was unfamiliar with commercially available bifurcated devices that would adequately seal a tapered 31 mm neck. The preoperative CT angiogram is seen in figure 3-12. After bilateral femoral arterial cutdown, a TAG endograft was placed in the left common iliac artery. Within this graft, two successfully larger TAG endografts were placed just below the renal arteries. Embolic coils were placed in the right internal iliac artery and the distal right external iliac artery was ligated. A femoral to femoral crossover graft with 8 mm ringed PTFE was constructed. The 75% left renal artery stenosis was repaired with angioplasty and stenting. Figure 3-13 illustrates the completed repair and figure 3-14 is the patient's postoperative

CT angiogram. The patient is alive over five years postoperatively with multiple hospitalizations secondary to pulmonary insufficiency. I believe this to be one of the first uses of a thoracic endograft in the abdominal aorta.

DISCUSSION OF AUI REPAIR

The AUI repair emerged early during the development of EVAR secondary to its ease of deployment and the availability of "homemade" devices. The AUI repair was particularly advantageous in the management of aneurysm rupture due to its simplicity and the avoidance of gate cannulation. The time saved by avoiding gate cannulation also reduces radiation exposure to both patient and surgeon. Preoperative sizing, in an emergency situation, is often not needed as the device can match virtually any patient with a proximal landing zone.

The most frequent indication for AUI repair is for patients with severe unilateral iliac occlusive disease. The initial fears that the femoral to femoral bypass component of the AUI would be prone to thrombosis have proved unfounded. Multiple studies have documented excellent patency rates for femoral crossover grafts when performed in conjunction with AUI repairs for aneurysmal disease.[8-10] In regards to preventing aneurysm rupture, both BF grafts and AUI grafts perform similarly.

COMMENTARY

(Scott L. Stevens, Knoxville, TN) This chapter details an innovative approach for treating complex aortic disease by constructing aorto-uniiliac (AUI) stent-grafts from available devices. The AUI evolution from homemade devices, to designing AUIs from available stents made for other positions to pathology specific, FDA approved AUIs is illustrated. Highlighted, is the broad perspective required to select the best therapy for these patients who present with demanding physiology and challenging vascular anatomy. All three case scenarios involve "off-label" use of stents and demonstrate the surgical creativity and courage required to explore all options and offer these patients the maximum benefit possible.

Key points in this chapter are the similar survival rates with bifurcated and AUI devices, the excellent patency of femoral crossover grafts, and the speed advantage of no gate cannulation when treating ruptured aneurysms.

REFERENCES

1. Parodi JC, Palmaz JC, Barone HD: Transfemoral intraluminal graft implantation for abdominal aortic aneurysms. *Ann Vasc Surg.* 1991; 5: 491-499.

2. Veith FJ: Emergency abdominal aortic aneurysm surgery. *Compr Ther.* 1992; 18: 25-29.

3. Yusuf SW, Whitaker SC, Chuter TA, et al. Emergency endovascular repair of leaking aortic aneurysms. *Lancet.* 1994; 344: 1645.

4. Ohki T, Veith FJ, Sanchez LA, et al. Endovascular graft repair of ruptured aorto-iliac aneurysm. *Am Coll Surg.* 1999; 189: 102-123.

5. Marin ML, Veith FJ, Cynamon J, et al. Initial experience with transluminally placed endovascular grafts for the treatment of complex vascular lesions. *Ann Surg.* 1995; 222: 1-17.

6. Veith FJ, Ohki T. Endovascular approaches – ruptured infrarenal aorto-iliac aneurysms. *J Cardiovasc Surg.* 2002; 43: 369-378.

7. Marin ML, Veith FJ. Endovascular stents and stented grafts for the treatment of aneurysm and other arterial lesions. *Adv Surg.* 1996; 29: 93-100.

8. Carpenter JP, Neschis DG, Fairman RM, et al. Failure of endovascular abdominal aortic aneurysm graft limbs. *J. Vasc Surg.* 2001; 33: 296-303.

9. Heredero AF, Stefanov S, Riera del Moral L, et al. Long-term results of femoral to femoral crossover bypass after endovascular aortouniiliac repair of abdominal aortic aneurysms. *Vasc and Endovasc Surg.* 2008; Vol 42:5, 420-426.

10. Riambau V, Hobo, R. Do bifurcated endografts produce better outcomes than aortouniiliac designs in endovascular aneurysm repair? *Hmp journals.* 2008; vol 5, (6) Nov/Dec.

11. Noorani A, Cooper DG, Walsh, SR, et al. Comparison of aortomonoiliac endovascular repair versus a bifurcated stent graft: Analysis of preoperative morbidity and mortality. *J Endovasc Ther.* 2009; 16: 295-301.

CHAPTER 4

Endovascular Repair of Acute Aortocaval Fistula

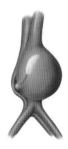

Aortocaval fistula (ACF) was first described by Syme in 1831.[1] Spontaneous ACFs are relatively rare and occur in less than 1% of all abdominal aortic aneurysms. However, when an ACF is found, it is associated with an abdominal aneurysm 80% of the time. The remaining 20% of ACFs are secondary to iatrogenic causes or other forms of trauma.[2-4] Approximately 50% of patients with ACF present with the classic triad of back pain, palpable abdominal mass, and abdominal bruit.[5] High output congestive heart failure, jugular venous distention, hepatomegaly, and leg edema are also common findings. Less likely findings include cyanosis, pulsating varicose veins, or priapism. Unfortunately many of these clinical signs mimic more common cardiac and renal abnormalities and diagnosis may be difficult without a high index of suspicion.[6] Prompt diagnosis is paramount as death from heart failure and cardiovascular collapse occurs within 24 hours of aortic rupture into the vena cava.[5-7]

An early successful surgical repair of a spontaneous ACF was described in 1954 by Cooley.[8] Even in recent series the operative mortality for the open surgical repair of ACFs is 30%.[5, 9, 10] Recently endovascular repairs of ACFs have been reported by a number of surgeons.[5-7, 11] In 2009 a systematic literature review of all English language journals identified only 22 patients with ACF treated by endovascular techniques. Sixty-five percent of these patients have primary spontaneous ACFs and 35% had secondary ACFs related to previous surgeries. The study further showed that 22% were misdiagnosed on initial presentation. Most importantly, the 30-day operative mortality for the endovascular treatment of ACFs was 0%. This is in stark contrast to the 30% mortality associated with open surgical repair.

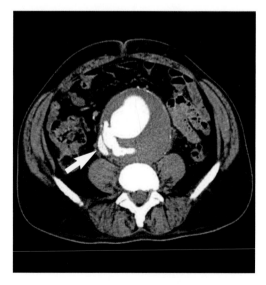

Figure 4-1 CT scan of 10.5 cm abdominal aortic aneurysm with rupture into the inferior vena cava. Note compression of cava, white arrow.

CASE SCENARIO:
Aortocaval Fistula

The patient is a 59-year-old man with a two and a half day history of fatigue, dyspnea, and mild ankle edema. His family physician noted an abdominal bruit and was suspicious of a cardiac etiology and referred the patient to the emergency department. A prompt CT scan demonstrated a 10.5 cm abdominal aortic aneurysm with rupture into the inferior vena cave, figure 4-1. The diagnosis had been made by the family physician and emergency room physician prior to consultation. The patient was taken urgently to the hybrid operating room. The intraoperative aortogram, figure 4-2, demonstrates a large abdominal aortic aneurysm with contrast dye rapidly filling the inferior vena cava. An illustration of the pathology is seen in figure 4-3. A bifurcated Excluder endograft was placed via the right femoral artery. Each limb received extension grafts. Intraoperative aortogram after graft placement demonstrated no endoleaks and no contrast flowing into the vena cava, figure 4-4. The left internal iliac artery was not embolized because there was thought to be an adequate "seal zone" on either side of the internal iliac. The patient did well postoperatively with almost immediate resolution of congestive heart failure symptoms, and was discharged home in a few days.

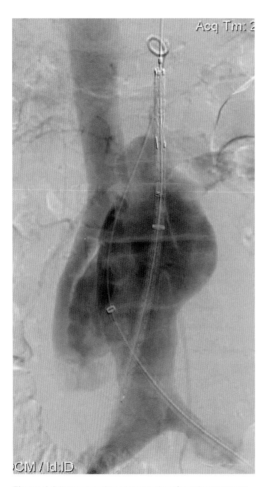

Figure 4-2 Intraoperative aortography of aortic aneurysm with rupture into the vena cava.

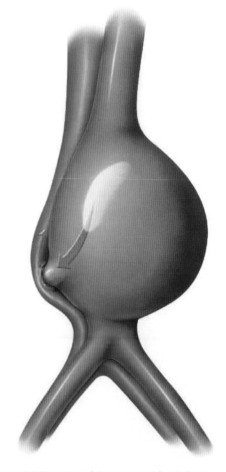

Figure 4-3 Illustration of the aortocaval fistula from aneurysm rupture.

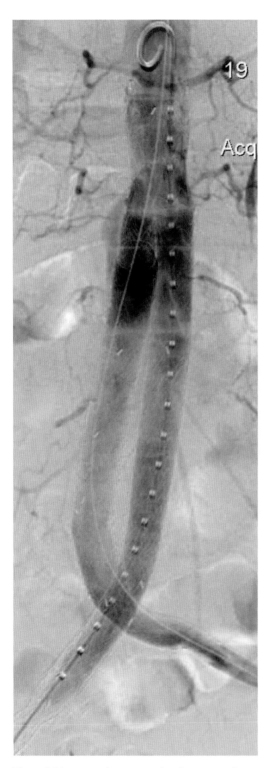

One-month postoperatively a CT angiogram demonstrated a small endoleak originating in the left internal iliac artery that tracked along the graft and ultimately emptied into the vena cava. The patient was asymptomatic and had a trivial nonphysiologic fistula. Little could be found in the literature regarding the management of this problem. Normally a small type-2 endoleak into a dead-end aneurysm sac would be of minimal clinical significance; however, if the type-2 leak could continuously empty into the low pressure cava, it would probably never seal. Could such a leak possibly enlarge over time?

The patient was returned to the operating room electively. A wire was navigated between the external iliac artery and the endograft to cannulate the internal iliac artery behind the endograft. Embolic coils were placed in the internal iliac artery, figure 4-5. Again no endoleaks could be detected by aortogram intraoperatively.

Two months after placing the coils, a CT angiography demonstrated a continued small endoleak ultimately emptying into the cava. Interestingly, the native aneurysm sac continued to decrease in size. Presumably, because the leak can empty into the vena cava, there is no endotension within the aneurysm sac. The patient continues to do well and is followed closely.

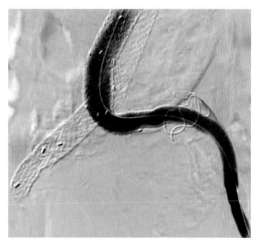

Figure 4-4 Intraoperative aortography after stent graft placement in ruptured aorta.

Figure 4-5 Arteriogram with embolic coils outside of the graft at origin internal iliac artery.

CASE DISCUSSION:
Aortocaval Fistula

The presence of an aortocaval fistula remains a rare event associated with less than 1% of all abdominal aortic aneurysms. Death is often sudden if not diagnosed promptly and a high index of suspicion is required. Open surgical intervention carries a 30% operative mortality. There was no operative mortality among the 22 reported cases corrected by endovascular techniques.[12] Although the endovascular repair of ACFs has a significant survival benefit versus open repair, it also is associated with those complications unique to endovascular surgery, such as endoleaks and residual fistulas as in the patient described.

The natural history of endoleaks in the setting of an ACF is unknown. It has been proposed that small endoleaks may be followed by annual vena cava duplex imaging and they may need no treatment at all.[4] At present, there are no long-term follow-up studies on the endovascular repair of ACFs and the rarity of the condition make multi-center controlled trials unlikely. One recent report describes placing a covered stent in the inferior vena cava to close a residual fistula.[13]

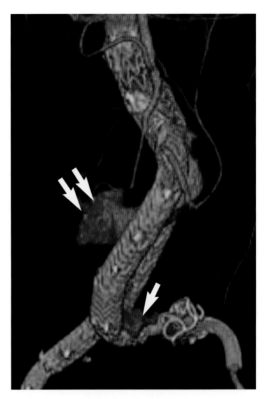

Figure 4-6 CT angiogram two months post initial procedure. Embolic coils in place but a small type 2 endoleak persists. Note: Contrast from left internal iliac (arrow) tracking along graft into AAA Sac (double arrow).

COMMENTARY

(Dennis R. Gable, Plano, TX) Chapter 4 demonstrates a very difficult and high risk problem that is seen only rarely in the practice of vascular surgery. The treatment offered to this patient as described throughout Chapter 4 offers an excellent chance for recovery and resolution of the patient's abdominal aortic aneurysm as well as the life threatening complication of an aorto-caval fistula. Although the data for this treatment is minimal due to the rarity of the disease process, the treatment option presented here offers a reasonable way for treatment of these patients and is rarely seen as an option outside of a large tertiary center.

REFERENCES

1. Syme J. Case of Spontaneous Varicose Aneurysm. *Edinberg Medical and Surgical Journal.* 1831; 36: 104-105.
2. David PM, Glovicski P, Cherry KJ. Aortocaval and Ilio-Iliac Arteriovenous Fistula: Rare and Challenging Problems. *American Journal of Surgery.* 1998; 176: 115.
3. Tsolakis JA, Papadoulas S, Kakkos SK, et al. Aortocaval Fistula in Ruptured Aneurysms. *European Journal of Vascular and Endovascular Surgery.* 17: 390-393.
4. Upchurch Jr GR, Criado E, eds. *Aortic Aneurysms Pathogenesis and Treatment.* Chapter 21. New York, NY: Humana Press; 2009.
5. Umscheid T Stelter. Endovascular Treatment of an Aortic Aneurysm Ruptured into the Inferior Vena Cava. *Journal of Endovascular Therapy.* 2000; 7: 31-35.
6. Lau LL, O'Reilly MJG, Johnston LC, et al. Endovascular Stent Graft Repair of Primary Aortocaval Fistula with an Abdominal Aortoiliac Aneurysm. *Journal of Vascular Surgery.* 2001; 33: 425-428.
7. Guzzardi G, Fossaceca R, Divenuto I, et al. Endovascular Treatment of Ruptured Abdominal Aortic Aneurysm with Aortocaval Fistula. *Cardiovascular Interventional Radiology.* 2010; 33: 853-856.
8. Cooley DA. Discussion of Paper by David and Coll: Resection of Ruptured Aneurysm of Abdominal Aorta. *Annals of Surgery.* 1955; 142: 623.
9. Beveridge CJ, Pleass HC, Chamberlain J, et al. Aortoiliac Aneurysm with Arteriocaval Fistula Treated with a Bifurcated Endovascular Stent Graft. *Cardiovascular Interventional Radiology.* 1998; 21: 244-246.
10. Fenster MS, Dent JM, Tribble C, et al. Aortocaval Fistula Complicating Abdominal Aortic Aneurysm: Case Report and Literature Review. *Catheterization and Cardiovascular Diagnosis.* 1996; 38: 75-79.
11. Vetrhus M, McWilliams R, Tan CK, et al. Endovascular Repair of Abdominal Aortic Aneurysms with Aortocaval Fistula. *European Journal of Vascular and Endovascular Surgery.* 2005; (30): 640-643.
12. Antoniou GA, Koutsias S, Karathomas C, et al. Endovascular Stent Graft Repair of Major Abdominal Arteriovenous Fistula: A Systematic Review. *Journal of Endovascular Therapy.* 2009; 16: 514-523.
13. Melas N, Athanasios S, Saratzis N, et al. Inferior Vena Cava Stent Graft Placement to Treat Endoleak Associated with Aortocaval Fistula. *Journal of Endovascular Therapy.* 2011; 18: 250-254.

CHAPTER 5

Endovascular Repair of a Ruptured Juxtarenal Paraanastomotic Aortic Aneurysm Utilizing Covered Chimney Stent Grafts for Renal Artery Rebranching

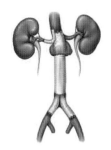

The prevalence of paraanastomotic aortic aneurysms (PAA) may be as high as 10%.[1-4] The incidence of PAA is known to increase over time and at 15 years post open aneurysm repair the incidence may be as high as 20%.[5] The incidence may actually be higher as most patients are asymptomatic and surveillance has not been routinely done for patients following open aneurysm repair. In addition, better general medical care and management of co morbidities has allowed patients to live longer following open aneurysmorrhaphy.

Elective open repair of PAA has a reported mortality of 4.5 to 17%, and emergency repair for rupture has a mortality approaching 70%.[5-7] The high mortality associated with this operation might be expected as the patients are often 10-15 years older and have developed other medical conditions since their original aneurysm surgery. In addition, the reoperative nature of the procedure and the management of the adjacent renal arteries contributes to an increase in mortality. Two studies have demonstrated that excluding the PAA with endovascular stent grafts have reduced the perioperative (30-day) mortality to 3.8%.[8, 9] However, the standard approach for endovascular repair of PAA required a region of relatively normal aorta below the renal arteries for graft

fixation even if a transrenal fixation strategy is employed. Many patients with juxtarenal PAA's do not have sufficient infrarenal aorta for adequate graft fixation. Such patients have been treated with customized fenestrated and branched endovascular stent grafts designed to preserve renal blood flow.[10-13] However, custom fenestrated grafts have not met current Food and Drug Administration approval in the United States and they are not readily available in emergency situations, such as in the event of rupture.

There are reports of preserving renal or mesenteric blood flood during the elective repair of PAA or with infrarenal aortic aneurysms with short necks by using "chimney grafts".[14-16] The following case report is believed to be the first report of total endovascular repair of a ruptured PAA using a covered Viabahn graft to preserve renal blood flow.

CASE SCENARIO:
Ruptured Paraanastomotic Aneurysm

An 87-year-old woman had undergone open repair of an infrarenal aortic aneurysm with a Dacron tube graft eleven years prior. She presented to the emergency department with back and flank pain.

Figures 5-1 and 5-2 demonstrate and illustrate the computerized tomographic (CT) findings of a ruptured 6.7 cm juxtrarenal paraanastomotic aortic aneurysm. The axillary artery was exposed by cutdown and a guidewire was placed in the right renal artery under fluoroscopic visualization. A long 60 cm 7-Fr destination sheath was positioned at the renal artery ostium and a 6 mm x 5 cm Viabahn covered graft was delivered partially within the renal artery, but not deployed. Bilateral femoral artery cutdowns were used to introduce and position a bifurcated Excluder endograft. The Excluder graft was positioned to cover or "over-stent" the origin of the native renal arteries. The covered renal graft was deployed as the main body of the Excluder was deployed, and they were balloon dilated simultaneously. The proximal extent of the covered renal graft was positioned to extend one-half of one centimeter above the main body of the Excluder. Figures 5-3 and 5-4 demonstrate and illustrate the completed procedure with exclusion of the aneurysm and no endoleaks. The patient remained endoleak free with no renal dysfunction at three month follow-up.

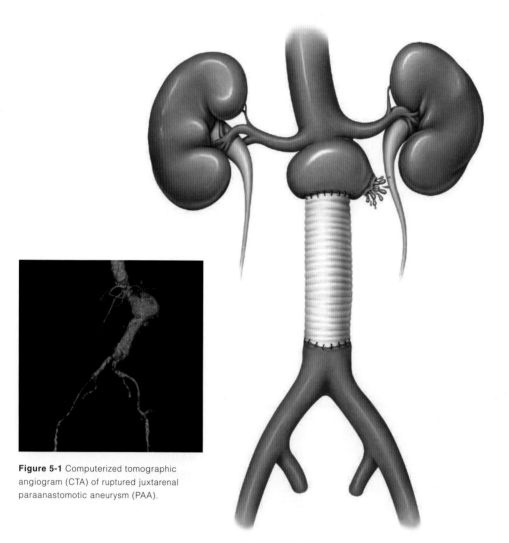

Figure 5-1 Computerized tomographic angiogram (CTA) of ruptured juxtarenal paraanastomotic aneurysm (PAA).

Figure 5-2 Illustration of ruptured juxtarenal PAA.

CASE DISCUSSION:
Ruptured Paraanastomotic Aneurysm

Juxtarenal PAA's increase in incidence with time from the initial surgery. The true incidence of PAA may be underestimated as open aneurysmorraphy has not been subjected to the surveillance scrutiny of endovascular procedures. The open surgical repair of juxtarenal PAA's has been associated with a high perioperative mortality for the reasons described earlier in this report. Endovascular repairs have a significantly lower mortality, but the lack of an adequate infrarenal aortic landing zone has eliminated some patients from endografting consideration. It is estimated that 20% of AAAs cannot be vented with currently approved EVAR devices. Customized fenestrated grafts are not readily available in the United States or in emergency situations. Chimney grafts may provide a viable alternative. This case scenario describes a successful endovascular repair of a "ruptured" juxtarenal PAA in an octogenarian using "off-the-shelf" components in a community hospital.

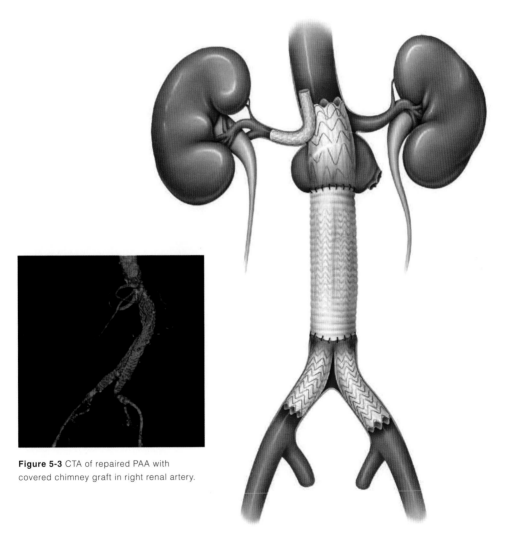

Figure 5-3 CTA of repaired PAA with covered chimney graft in right renal artery.

Figure 5-4 Illustration of repaired ruptured PAA with covered chimney graft in right renal artery.

COMMENTARY

(Scott L. Stevens, Knoxville, TN) Open repair of paraanstomotic aneurysms (PAAs) requires dissection through scarred tissue planes in a high-stakes locale. As outlined in this chapter, surgical correction of these PAAs is technically demanding and incurs high perioperative morbidity and mortality. This case scenario clearly illustrates an innovative solution to a complex, lethal problem – a ruptured juxtarenal aortic aneurysm. Snorkels, chimneys, periscopes and even "hot dog in a bun" are all terms coined to describe the technique of extending a stent-graft landing zone past critical side branches by using parallel stent grafts. This case represents an elegant strategy that uses brachial and femoral access to maintain parallel conduits for renal perfusion and aortic stent graft exclusion of the aortic rupture. The lifesaving and pioneering efforts, exemplified in this chapter, will soon be eclipsed with commercially made grafts constructed with side branches and fenestrations.

REFERENCES

1. James M, Eduardo MD, Sharlene A, Teefey MD, et al. Intraabdominal Paraanastomotic Aneurysms After Aortic Bypass Grafting. *Journal of Vascular Surgery*. 1992; 15: 344-353.
2. Plate G, Hollier LA, O'Brien P, et al. Recurrent Aneurysms and Late Vascular Complications Following Repair of Abdominal Aortic Aneurysms. *Archives of Surgery*. 1985; 120: 590-594.
3. Sieswerda C, Skotnicki SH, Barentsz JO, et al. Anastomotic Aneurysms – A Underdiagnosed Complication After Aortoiliac Reconstructions. *European Journal of Vascular Surgery*. 1998; 3: 233-23.
4. Dennis JEWY, Littooy FN, Greister HP, et al. Anastamotic Pseudoaneurysms: A Continuing Late Complication of Vascular Reconstructive Procedures. *Archives of Surgery*. 1986; 121: 314-317.
5. Mulder EJ, VanBockel H, Maas J, et al. Morbidity and Mortality of Reconstructive Surgery of Noninfected False Aneurysms Detected After Aortic Prosthetic Reconstruction. *Archives of Surgery*. 1998; 133: 45-49.
6. Allen RC, Schneider J, Longenecker L, et al. Paraanastomotic Aneurysms of the Abdominal Aorta. *Journal of Vascular Surgery*. 1993; 18: 424-431; Discussion 431-432.
7. Curl GR, Faggioli GL, Stella A, et al. Aneurysmal Change at or Above the Proximal Anastomosis After Infrarenal Aortic Grafting. *Journal of Vascular Surgery*. 1992; 16: 855-859; Discussion 859-860.
8. Morrissey NJ, Yano OH, Soundararajen K., et al. Endovascular Repair of Paraanastomotic Aneuryms of the Aorta and Iliac Arteries: Preferred Treatment For a Complex Problem." *Journal of Vascular Surgery*. 2001; 33: 503-512.
9. Sachder U, Baril DT, Morrissey NJ, et al. Endovascular Repair of Paraanastomotic Aortic Aneurysms. *Journal of Vascular Surgery*. 2007; 36: 636-641
10. Greenberg RK, Haulon S, O'Neills, et al. Primary Endovascular Repair of Juxtrarenal Aneurysms with Fenestrated Endovascular Grafting. *European Journal of Vascular and Endovascular Surgery*. 2004; 27: 484-491.
11. Greenberg RK, Haulon S, Lyden SP, et al. Endovascular Management of Juxtarenal Aneurysms With Fenestrated Endovascular Grafting. *Journal of Vascular Surgery*. 2004; 39: 279-287.
12. Adam DJ, Berce M, Hartley DE and Anderson JO. Repair of Juxtrarenal Paraanastomotic Aneurysms After Previous Open Repair With Fenestrated and Branched Endovascular Stent Grafts. *Journal of Vascular Surgery*. 2005; 42: 997-1001.
13. Verhoeven ELG, Prins TR, Tielliu IFJ, et al. Treatment of Short-Necked Infrarenal Aortic Aneurysms With Fenestrated Stent Grafts: Short-Term Results. *European Journal of Vascular and Endovascular Surgery*. 2004; 27y: 477-483.
14. Ohrlander T, Sonesson B, Ivancev K, et al. The Chimney Graft: A Technique For Preserving or Rescuing Aortic Branch Vessels In Stent-Graft Sealing Zones. *Journal of Endovascular Therapy*. 2008; 15: 427-432.
15. Criado FJ. Chimney Grafts and Bare Stents. *Journal of Endovascular Therapy*. 2007; 14: 823-824.
16. Criado FJ. Conquering Zone Zero: Expanding Endograft Repair In the Aortic Arch. *Journal of Endovascular Therapy*. 2008; 15: 166-167.

CHAPTER 6

Endovascular Repair of a Juxtarenal Abdominal Aortic Aneurysm Using Chimney Grafts for Renal Artery Preservation

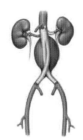

Endograft repair of aortic aneurysms requires an adequate landing zone for endograft fixation both proximally and distally. Limitations in landing zones involve size constraints, circumferential thrombus, severe neck angulation, and the presence of arterial side branches. Size constraints are landing zones that are either too large or too narrow to allow for endograft fixation. If thrombus circumferentially lines the inner wall of the landing zone, endograft fixation may be compromised leading to endoleak or endograft migration. Extreme neck angulation may lead to graft migration due to a decrease in the effective length of the landing zone. In addition, the sidewall and flow divider of an angulated graft will contribute to migration.

Finally, the location of aortic side branch arteries can effectively limit the length of available landing zones. Side branch preservation and revascularization has been reported with the use of Chimney Grafts; also called parallel, snorkel, or double-barrel grafts.[1-8] As mentioned in Chapter 5, custom factory-made branched endografts are available in some countries; although they are not yet approved for use in the United States. In addition, these custom factory-made grafts are constructed as ordered for individual patients and are therefore not readily available in an emergency situation.

The case scenario below describes a patient

with impaired renal function, a large symptomatic juxtarenal aortic aneurysm, and an inadequate proximal landing zone.

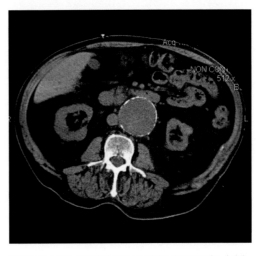

Figure 6-1 Non-contrast computerized tomography. Axial view.

CASE SCENARIO:
Renal Artery Chimney Grafts

The patient is a 76 year-old man transferred from an outside hospital with new onset severe back pain, a 6.8 cm juxtarenal aortic aneurysm, and a stage-4 kidney disease with a baseline creatinine of 3.2 mg/dl. The patient has been under the care of a

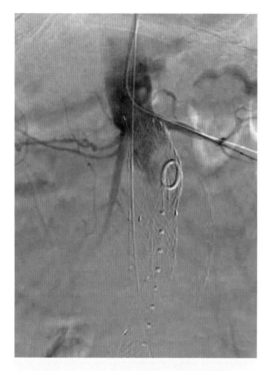

Figure 6-2 Intraoperative arteriogram post deployment of main graft and left renal artery chimney graft. Note wire in left renal artery via axillary artery.

nephrologist and it was believed he would require permanent dialysis for deteriorating renal function within the next 6 to 12 months. The non-contrast CT demonstrated a 6.8 cm aneurysm, a small right renal artery, and a normal size left renal artery, figure 6-1.

The patient was not deemed to be an open-surgical candidate due to comorbidities and standard endografting techniques would occlude the origin of both renal arteries. Endografting to intentionally occlude the renal arteries was considered as the patient would ultimately require dialysis in his lifetime regardless of treatment modality.

However, a third option would be to place a Chimney Graft in the larger left renal artery to perfuse the left kidney while covering, or over-stenting both native renal ostia with an endograft. If successful, this would treat the aneurysm and potentially allow the patient to live another year or more without the burden of dialysis. If in the event a proximal type-I endoleak develops, a

cuff-extender could be used to seal the leak and obliterate the Chimney Graft. In that scenario, the patient would be no worse off than if the renal arteries had been covered initially, and he would at least have been given the change to avoid dialysis for possibly another year.

Under general anesthesia, bilateral femoral and left axillary artery cutdowns were performed. Via the left axillary artery, the left renal artery was cannulated with 0.018 inch wire. This was subsequently changed to an 0.035 inch wire and a 7-Fr 60 cm sheath was positioned at the origin of the left renal artery. A 6 mm by 5 cm viabahn covered stent graft was positioned but not deployed in the left renal artery. An Excluder bifurcated endograft was placed with the main body via the right femoral artery.

The intrarenal portion (distal 2.5-3 cm) of the Viabahn graft was expanded, then the main body of the endograft was deployed. Finally, the distal one-half of the Viabahn graft was deployed so that it extended one-half to one centimeter above the main body of the Excluder graft. Figure 6-2 is the intraoperative post procedure arteriogram demonstrating no endoleak, correction of the aneurysm, preservation of flow through the chimney graft to the left renal artery, and no compromise of flow in the superior mesenteric artery. A total of 40 ml of contrast as administered during the procedure. The patient was discharged home with a stable baseline creatinine and has remained dialysis free for 13 months following the procedure.

Figure 6-3 illustrates the relationship of the main graft to the left renal chimney. A computerized tomographic scan without contrast demonstrates the orientation of the bifurcated endograft with respect to the left renal chimney graft, figure 6-4. Note the calcified outline of the large aneurysms sac. As will be discussed in Chapter 8, Chimney grafts seldom make a 90 degree turn as they exit a side branch; rather they tend to "spiral" alongside the main body graft. This makes underestimating the necessary length of the chimney a potential error.

CASE DISCUSSION

It is estimated that 20% of AAAs are not treatable by currently approved EVAR devices. Also, custom-made fenestrated grafts are still awaiting FDA approval. In situations, such as the patient presented, chimney grafts may serve as a viable alternative.

Current trials are underway with the Ventana graft (Endologix Corp., Irvine, CA). The Ventana graft is intended to be an off-the-shelf endograft to treat Juxtarenal AAAs. The Ventana graft has a scalloped upper section to allow for mesenteric perfusion and covered grafts for the renal arteries, see Chapter 23.

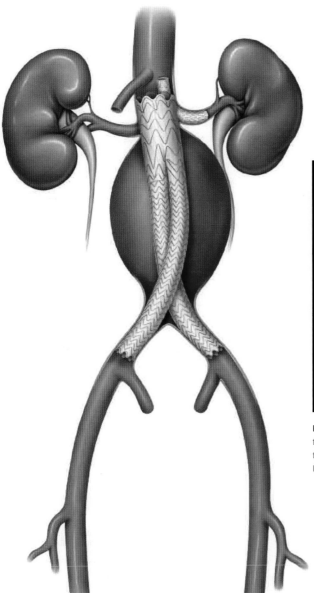

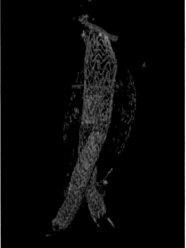

Figure 6-4 Non-contrast computerized tomography. Note relation of chimney graft to main body graft and calcium outline of large aneurysm sac.

Figure 6-3 Illustration of chimney graft in left renal artery.

COMMENTARY

(Dennis R. Gable, Plano, TX) The case presented in Chapter 6 provides a more recent available option for treatment of patients that have a short landing zone for the proximal portion of an aortic endograft when treating aortic aneurismal disease. This technique is typically something reserved for use in large university centers and is rarely used in the smaller community setting. In fact, this is a good option for these patients and offers the availability of endovascular treatment rather than open surgical repair thus decreasing the complications that can ensue with open surgical aneurismal repair.

REFERENCES

1. Baldwin ZK, Chuter TAM, Hiramoto JS, et al. Double-Barrel Techniques for Exclusion of an Aortic Arch Aneurysm Without Sternotomy. *Journal of Endovascular Therapy.* 2008; 15: 161-165.

2. Ohrlander T, Sonesson, B, Ivancev K, et al. The Chimney Graft: A Technique for Preserving or Rescuing Aortic Branch Vessels in Stent-Graft Sealing Zones. *Journal of Endovascular Therapy.* 2008; 15: 427-432.

3. Baldwin ZK, Chuter TAM, Hiramoto JS, et al. Double-Barrel Techniques for Preservation of Aortic Arch Branches During Thoracic Endovascular Aortic Repair. *Annals of Vascular Surgery.* 2008; 22: 703-709.

4. Hiramoto JS, Schneider DB, Reilly LM, et al. A Double-Barrel Stent-Graft for Endovascular Repair of Aortic Arch. *Journal of Endovascular Therapy.* 2006; 13: 72-76.

5. Kristmundsson T, Sonesson B, Malina M, et al. Fenestrated Endovascular Repair for Juxtarenal Aortic Pathology. *Journal of Vascular Surgery.* 2009; In Press.

6. Adam DJ, Berce M, Hartley D, et al. Repair of Juxtarenal Para-Anastomotic Aortic Aneurysms After Previous Open Repair With Fenestrated and Branched Endovascular Stent Grafts. *Journal of Vascular Surgery.* 2005; 42: 997-1001.

7. Criado FJ. Chimney Grafts and Bare Stents. *Journal of Endovascular Therapy.* 2007; 14: 823-824.

8. Criado FJ. Conquering Zone Zero: Expanding Endograft Repair in the Aortic Arch. *Journal of Endovascular Therapy.* 2008; 15: 166-167.

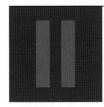

SECTION II

Thoracic and Thoracoabdominal Aortic Aneurysms

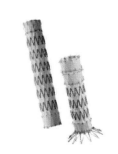

CHAPTER 7

Thoracic Aortic Aneurysms: Etiology, Natural History, and Thoracic Endografts

The thoracic aorta is susceptible to a variety of pathologies including: trauma, aneurysm, dissection, connective tissue disorders, penetrating ulcers, and intramural hemorrhage. These maladies may be distinct or occur as part of a spectrum of aortic disease. For example, either a penetrating ulcer or Marfan syndrome can lead to aortic dissection which subsequently can enlarge and become an aortic aneurysm. Among all aortic aneurysms, 80% are confined to the abdominal aorta and 20% occur within the thoracic or thoracoabdominal aorta. Thoracic aortic aneurysms (TAAs) can occur in any section of the thoracic aorta and those extending into the abdomen are called thoracoabdominal aortic aneurysms (TAAAs). Figure 7-1 illustrates the relative percentage of thoracic aneurysm occurrence by aortic segment.[1] This chapter will focus on aneurysms that originate at or distal to the left subclavian artery.

ETIOLOGY OF THORACIC AORTIC ANEURYSMS

The majority of TAAs are the result of medial degeneration within the wall of the aorta. Medial degeneration is the new terminology for what was once called cystic medial necrosis. Medial degeneration is multifactorial and involves a

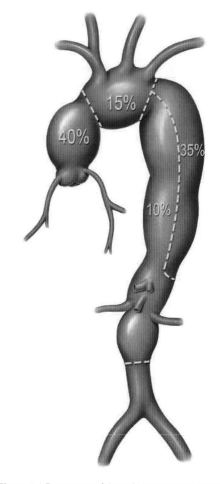

Figure 7-1 Percentage of thoracic aneurysm occurrence by segment of the aorta.

complex interplay between hemodynamic forces, genetic factors, and matrix metalloproteinases (MMPs). The final product of this interaction is the breakdown of the extracellular matrix (ECM) and the smooth muscle cell components within the aortic wall. The ECM is composed of actin, myosin, collagen, and elastin. The different segments of the aorta have varying percentages of the ECM components. The elastin to collagen ratio within the aortic wall decreases as one progresses from the proximal to distal aorta. Thus, the ascending aorta has the highest elastin to collagen ratio and elastin confers more compliance to the aortic tissue.[4, 5] Although hemodynamic forces are certainly involved, the increased elastin in the ascending aorta may explain the observation that aneurysms of the ascending aorta expand at a faster rate than aneurysms of the descending thoracic aorta.

Although the majority of TAAs are the result of medial degeneration, is estimated the 20% to 50% of TAAs arise in an area of previous aortic dissection.[6-10] However, the dissection itself was probably the result of medial degeneration. Whereas it may be easy to discern an aneurysm versus dissection based on radiographic or intraoperative findings, I believe that on the cellular and macromolecular level, aneurysms and dissections are a part of a spectrum of the same disease.

GENETIC FACTORS AND TAAs

TAAs and thoracic acute aortic dissections (TAADs) have been classified as syndromic, familial, or sporadic. Syndromic TAAs occur as part of a syndrome of clinical manifestations such as Marfan syndrome (MFS), Ehlers-Danlos type-IV syndrome (EDS), or Loeys-Dietz syndrome (LDS). Less than 5% of TAAS are classified as syndromic. Generally a specific genetic defect is identified in patients with syndromic TAAs. Familial TAAs represent 15% to 20% of TAAs. A number of specific gene mutations have been identified in families with TAAs in their pedigrees. Eighty percent of TAAs are classified as sporadic. Although

this group is classified as sporadic because there is not a clustering of first of second degree relatives with TAAs in the family pedigree, it does not mean that there is not a specific genetic defect responsible for their aneurysms. Indeed many patients having what is classified as a sporadic or randomly occurring TAA, have now been identified as carrying specific genetic mutations that occur more frequently in TAA patients than in the general population.

SYNDROMIC TAAs (3%-5%)

The syndromic group of TAAs includes Marfan (MFS), Ehlers-Danlos – IV (EDS), Loeys-Dietz (LDS) syndrome.

Marfan Syndrome

MFS is an connective tissue disorder with autosomal dominant inheritance that occurs with an incidence of 1 in 10,000 individuals. Affected patients display varying degrees of dolichostenomelia, ectopia lentis, arachnodactyly, and TAAs. The underlying defect in MFS is a mutation in the fibrillin-1 (FBN1) gene.[11, 12] Nearly 600 mutations of the FBN1 gene have been identified. Because of the many different mutated forms of the FBN1 gene and the fact that 25% of patients have a de novo mutation, the role of genetic screening to diagnose this disease is limited. Currently clinical manifestations are the mainstay of diagnosing MFS. Type A aortic dissections are the most common cause of death in patients with MFS. Aortic root replacement should be performed prophylactically with an ascending aortic diameter of 5 cm or sooner with the development of concurrent aortic valvular insufficiency. In the 1970s, the life expectancy of patient with MFS was reported as two-thirds that of the unaffected population. Recent reports demonstrate that patients with MFS have a nearly normal life expectancy as a result of improved diagnosis and surgical management of the aortic root pathology.[13-15]

Ehlers-Danlos IV Syndrome

Ehlers-Danlos (EDS) syndrome is a disorder characterized by tissue fragility of the skin, joints, internal organs, and blood vessels. Specifically EDS type IV is associated with the vascular manifestations of rupture and dissection. EDS IV is inherited in an autosomal dominant fashion and occurs with an incidence of 1 in 50,000 population.[16] Affected patients have a mutation in the COL3A1 gene which encodes for type-III procollagen.[17, 18] The procollagen alpha chains cannot fold into a stable triple helix and thus are degraded within the cell as opposed to their normal pathway of being secreted into the ECM. The median life expectancy of patients with EDS IV is 48 years with 60% of the deaths attributed to vascular rupture.[19] Interestingly, the arterial rupture or dissection occurs most commonly in medium sized arteries of the chest and abdomen as opposed to the aorta itself. This is in contradistinction to MFS patients in which the aorta is the most commonly affected artery.

The open surgical management of arterial rupture in patients with EDS is fraught with bleeding secondary to tissue fragility. Because of the fragile nature of the arteries in these patients, vessel ligation or coil embolization is employed whenever possible. Diagnosis should be made by CT angiography. Percutaneous arterial puncture should be avoided. If intraarterial diagnostic studies or arterial embolization are required, the access artery should be approached by open cutdown so that it can be surgically repaired. One study documents a 67% major complication rate and a 12% mortality rate from attempts at percutaneous arterial access in EDS patients.[20]

Loeys-Dietz Syndrome

Loeys-Dietz syndrome (LDS) is characterized by the clinical manifestations of a cleft palate or bifid uvula, hypertelorism, and retrognathia. LDS is caused by missense mutations in the transforming growth factor-B1 and 2 receptors (TGFBR1 and TGFBR2). Affected patients develop extremely tortuous and aneurysmal aortas at a very young age. Prophylactic aortic root replacement should be considered at a diameter of 4 cm.

An overriding principal for patients with connective tissue disorders is early diagnosis, surveillance and open surgery if needed. Endovascular stent grafts should be generally avoided. The fragility of the aortic tissue renders endograft landing zones and fixation suspect at best. Additionally, the long-term outward radial force of the endograft against the weakened aortic wall may cause further aortic injury. Rarely, in an emergency situation, endografts may be used in patients with connective tissue disorders as a "bridge" until a time when a more definitive procedure can be performed.

FAMILIAL TAAs (15% TO 20%)

Approximately 15% to 20% of patients with a TAA have a first degree relative with a TAA.[21, 22] Although these TAAs cluster in families and would clearly have a genetic component, they are not associated with a syndrome such as MFS, EDS, or LDS. In most families with TAAs, the disorder is inherited in an autosomal dominant manner with decreased penetrance and variable expression with respect to the age of onset of aortic dilatation.[18] In general, patients with familial TAAs present at a younger age than patients with sporadic TAAs. Some families with TAAs have an associated bicuspid aortic valve. Other families have TAAs and an associated patent ductus arteriosus. These associations may be part of a specific genetic defect; however, they do not classify as syndromic TAAs. The primary causative genes associated with familial TAAs are ACTA2, TGFBR2, and MYH11. ACTA2 mutations may be responsible for 10% to 14% of familial TAAs.

SPORADIC TAAs (80%)

Nearly 80% of patients with TAAs are classified as having sporadic or random TAAs. These patients are not identified with a syndrome and they do not have family members with TAAs in their pedigree. However, they still may have a genetic basis for their disease that has not been fully elucidated. One report documented chromosome duplications in the 16p13.1 region are associated with the development of TAAs. Duplications of chromosome 16p13.1 were found in 1% of patients with adult onset sporadic TAAs and in 0.09% of the general population. Thus, a person has a 12-fold increased risk of having a TAA if they have chromosome 16p13.1 duplication.[23] A likely gene culprit is MYH11, which resides in the 16p13.1 region and codes for the smooth muscle cell specific B-myosin heavy chain isoform. Defects in this gene would weaken the smooth muscle component of the extracellular matrix; a recurring theme in aortic disease.

TAA INCIDENCE AND RISK OF RUPTURE

Thoracic aortic aneurysms have an incidence of 6 per 100,000 patient-years. The incidence of a ruptured TAA is 3.5 to 5 per 100,000 patient-years, with an overall risk of rupture in a 5 year period of 20%.[6-8] The risk of rupture for a given size TAA in women is seven times that of men. Although not as well-defined as for abdominal aortic aneurysm, TAAs also display an increasing risk of rupture with increasing size and that risk rises significantly with a diameter great than 6 cm.[24] Thoracoabdominal aortic aneurysms (TAAAs) with a diameter greater than or equal to 8 cm have an 80% risk of rupture within 1 year of diagnosis.[25] In a study of 170 patients with TAAs, AAAs and TAAAs who did not undergo surgery; the 5-year overall survival was 39% for patients with TAAs, 23% for patients with TAAAs and 18% for patients with AAAs.[26, 27]

OPEN REPAIR OF TAAs

The open surgical repair of TAAs has always been associated with a significant operative mortality. In the text by Stevens and Farber, they reviewed multiple reports containing over 1,600 patients undergoing elective open repair for descending TAAs. The mean 30-day mortality was 9.2% with a range of 4.4% to 31%.[27] The National Inpatient Sample Administrative Database, which likely reflects broad-based real-world experience, reports an operative mortality of 10% for all elective descending TAA repairs and a mortality of 45% for all repairs of ruptured descending TAAs.[28] The Baylor group reported 387 patients undergoing open repair of TAAs with a mortality of 4.4%, paraplegia 2.6%, stroke 1.8% and renal failure 7.5%.[29] The Baylor report may represent the best results that can be attained, but even in the best of hands at high-volume centers, the open repair of TAAs is accompanied by a significant risk of death and complication.

THORACIC ENDOGRAFTS
GORE – TAG Graft 2005

The TAG endograft is essentially a tube of expanded PTFE with a nitinol exoskeleton. The nitinol is fixed to the PTFE with banding tape constructed from PTFE, figure 7-2. The device is delivered on a 100 cm flexible delivery catheter with a tapered bead or "olive" on each end of the catheter. The tapered "olive" theoretically allows for less traumatic passage of the catheter in the aorta. Also the tapered end makes it easier to pass one ELG inside another ELG when 2 or more grafts are needed. Deployment of the TAG differs from most endografts and consists of pulling a "delivery line." Pulling the "delivery line" initiates expansion of the TAG graft, starting in the middle of the graft and progressing to each end. A unique trilobed balloon can be inflated within the graft to more tightly appose the graft to the aortic wall. The trilobed design allows for the balloon to contact and expand the graft while also allowing blood to flow between the lobes. Theoretically this minimizes the chance that the pressure of aortic blood flow will cause the inflated balloon to "bounce" distally and move the graft along with it.

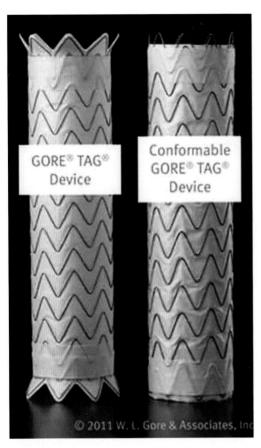

Figure 7-2 GORE TAG thoracic endoprosthesis (left) and GORE Conformable CTAG thoracic endoprosthesis (right). Image courtesy W.L. Gore and Associates. Flagstaff, AZ.

GORE Pivotal Phase II (TAG) Trial

The pivotal trial was a multicenter study designed to determine the effectiveness and safety of the TAG graft by comparison to open surgery for the treatment of descending TAAs. The study was conducted at 17 clinical sites between 1999 and 2001. One hundred and forty patients were initially selected for the TAG ELG arm and 94 patients served as the control group for open surgery. Operative (30-day) mortality occurred in 2.1% of the endograft group and in 11.7% of the open surgical cohort. Paralysis or paraplegia occurred in 3% of the endograft group versus 13.7% in the open surgical group.[30] In addition, ICU stay, hospital stay, and blood transfusion requirements were

significantly lower in the TAG group. The Gore TAG device gained FDA approval in March 2005.

The newer generation Conformable TAG (C-TAG) is expected to be released for general use in October 2011. The manufacturer reports the device to be conformable and compression resistant in 33% over sizing conditions. The C-TAG has uncovered proximal flares, thicker nitinol wires, a ninth apex to proximal stent pattern, and the smallest available graft diameter at 21 mm, figure 7-2. Because of the "compression resistance" the manufacturer indicates the smallest diameter C-TAG (21 mm) can be placed in a 16 mm diameter aorta. Although the C-TAG is not in general use at the time of writing this chapter, I discuss its use in the patient presented in Chapter 21.

Medtronic Talent Graft 2008

The Talent endograft is a Dacron polyester tube sutured to a self-expanding nitinol wire frame. Diameters varied between 22 mm to 46 mm with a maximal total length of 130 mm, figure 7-3. The graft was initially deployed with a push rod in the CoilTrac delivery system. The recent version of the Talent graft uses the Captivia delivery system. The Captivia system is more flexible than the CoilTrac and has a hydrophilic outer coating. Post deployment, a balloon can be used to expand the graft fabric and further appose the Talent ELG to the aortic wall. The Talent graft had been used successfully in nearly 1,000 patients outside of the United States prior to receiving FDA approval following the VALOR Trial.

Medtronic VALOR (Talent) Trial

The VALOR trial was a prospective non randomized, multicenter trial conducted at 38 clinical sites. The trial was designed to determine the effectiveness and safety of the Talent thoracic endoprosthesis for treating descending TAAs and penetrating ulcers by comparison with retrospective open surgical controls from three centers of excellence. The study enrolled 195

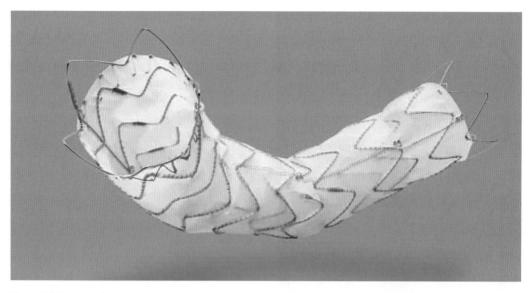

Figure 7-3 Medtronic Talent thoracic endoprosthesis. Image courtesy of Medtronic Inc., Santa Rosa, CA.

patients from December 2003 until June 2005. All cause mortality was significantly reduced in the endograft arm versus the open surgery arm (2.1% vs. 7.9%, P<0.01). Also the 12-month aneurysm-related mortality was less in the Talent group versus open group (3.1% vs. 11.6%, P<0.002). Paraplegia occurred in only 1.5% of the endograft cohort. No instances of aortic perforation occurred during Talent graft deployment.[31] The VALOR trail demonstrated the Talent graft to be a safe and effective therapy for descending TAAs. The FDA gave approval for the Talent thoracic stent graft on June 5, 2008.

Medtronic Valiant Graft 2011

The Valiant thoracic endoprosthesis is the latest generation Medtronic graft approved for use in the United States. The Valiant stent graft is essentially a new and improved Talent stent graft with changes made over 10 years of worldwide clinical experience with the Talent graft. The nitinol wires of the Valiant graft are slightly thicker at 0.021-inches and sutured to the outside of the graft. There are 8 spring peaks on the Valiant graft as opposed to 5 with the Talent graft, figure 7-4. Also the removal of

the connecting bar, found on the Talent device, allows the Valiant graft to be positioned without concern for in vivo orientation. One would intuitively think that by not needing to rotate or orient the graft within the aorta that the risk of embolic stroke would decrease. Another advantage with the Valiant graft is that it comes in longer (220 mm)

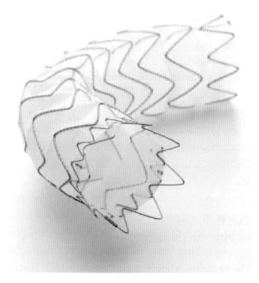

Figure 7-4 Medtronic Valiant thoracic endoprosthesis. Image courtesy of Medtronic Corp., Santa Rosa, CA.

lengths than did the Talent graft (130 mm). Most aortic pathology requires a graft longer than 130 mm. Longer grafts mean fewer device manipulations in the aorta which could reduce the incidence of stroke. Also, fewer passes through the iliac arteries would reduce the chance of iliac artery injury. The Captivia delivery system allows for the controlled release of the proximal portion of the graft to prevent the "windsock" effect.

The VALOR II trial enrolled 160 patients between December 2006 and September 2009 at 24 clinical sites in the United States. At 12 months follow-up, aneurysm-related death in the endograft group was 3.3%. The FDA approved the Valiant stent graft for use in the United States on April 1, 2011.

Cook Zenith TX2 2008

The Zenith TX2 thoracic endograft is a tubular Dacron stent graft supported by stainless steel stents. This is in contradistinction to the other approved thoracic grafts which employ nitinol stents. The Zenith TX2 graft is constructed with the Dacron fabric on the outside of the stainless steel stents proximally and distally, figure 7-5. However, the midportion of the graft has the fabric on the inside of the stents. The Zenith device can function as a 1-piece graft but is primarily designed as a 2-piece system. The proximal portion has a series of 5 mm caudally-oriented barbs to prevent distal migration. The distal component has a series of cranially-oriented bars to prevent proximal migration. Although only time will tell, the stainless steel skeleton would be expected to have a durability advantage over a nitinol skeleton. The Valiant thoracic graft received FDA approval May 21, 2008.

CASE SCENARIO:
TEVAR for Descending TAA

The patient is a 66-year-old woman with a 5.3 cm descending TAA referred for surgical consideration. Three years prior an MRA scan had demon-

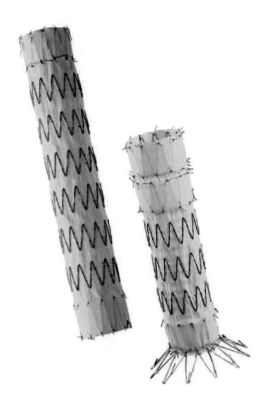

Figure 7-5 Cook Zenith TX2 thoracic endoprosthesis. Proximal component (left), distal component (right). Image courtesy of Cook Medical, Bloomington, IN.

strated the TAA to be 4.5 cm in diameter, figure 7-6. During the preoperative preparation for TEVAR the patient was diagnosed with significant left main coronary artery disease and I performed routine 2-vessel coronary bypass grafting with the use of the left internal mammary artery as an in situ conduit.

Fourteen days after the coronary bypass procedure, TEVAR was schedule. The right common femoral artery was exposed by cutdown and a 0.035-inch soft guidewire was positioned in the ascending aorta with fluoroscopic visualization. The soft wire was exchanged to a stiff Lunderquist wire by use of a guide catheter. A 22-Fr sheath was delivered over the Lunderquist wire and positioned in the abdominal aorta. The left common femoral artery was cannulated by percutaneous puncture

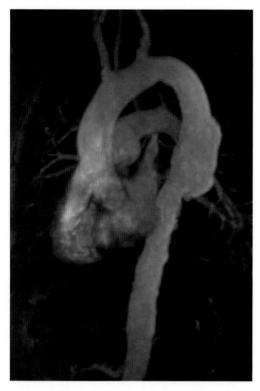

Figure 7-6 Magnetic resonance angiogram of small descending TAA three years before repair.

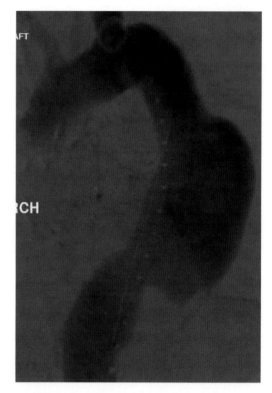

Figure 7-7 Intraoperative aortagram prior to ELG placement.

and used to introduce a pigtail marking catheter into the ascending aorta. An intraoperative aortogram demonstrating the descending TAA is seen in figure 7-7. The TAA was repaired with 2 TAG ELGs sizes 31 mm by 15 cm and 31 mm by 10 cm. The junctures were expanded to contour with a trilobed balloon. The completion aortogram demonstrates exclusion of the TAA with no evidence of endoleak, figure 7-8. The surveillance CT angiogram 2 years following the procedure is seen in figure 7-9.

CASE DISCUSSION:
TEVAR for Descending TAA

This case describes the routine and uneventful TEVAR of a descending TAA; yet a number of issues merit discussion concerning TEVAR in general and in regards to this case in particular.

First, TEVAR is a significantly safer and less morbid procedure than the open surgical repair of descending TAAs. Three major trials evaluating the TAG, Talent, and Zenith TX2 endografts all confirm a 30 day operative mortality for TEVAR between 2% to 3.5%. The average nationwide mortality for open TAA repair approaches 10% and the high-volume specialized centers report a mortality of 4.4%. Also, paralysis rates for TEVAR are approximately 3% versus 10% to 13% for open TAA repair. The mere fact that the case described was so "uneventful" is a testament to the technological advantage of TEVAR.

For the specific patient presented, the patient was a woman. Although all types of aortic aneurysms occur more frequently in men than in women, women comprise a relatively higher percentage of TAA patients than AAA patients. Also, the patient in our care did not require an iliac

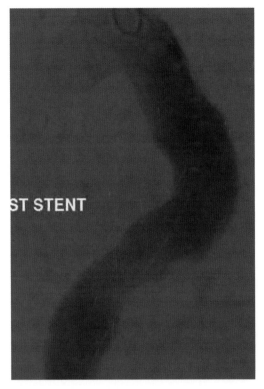

Figure 7-8 Intraoperative aortogram post ELG placement.

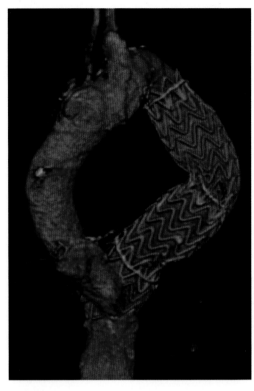

Figure 7-9 CT angiogram 2 years post TEVAR demonstrating successful TAA exclusion.

artery conduit for endograft delivery; 20% of patients do require a conduit for TEVAR.

In addition, this patient did not require coverage of the left subclavian artery (LSCA) to adequately repair her TAA. If coverage of the LSCA is necessary, then a left carotid artery to LSCA bypass may or may not be required. Coverage of the LSCA will obstruct blood flow in the left vertebral artery and potentially cause vertebrobasilar insufficiency or a vertebrobasilar stroke. Fortunately, 97% of patients have a dominant right vertebral artery and occlusion of the LSCA (and left vertebral) may be tolerated. If longer segments of the thoracic or thoracoabdominal aorta are expected to be covered with an ELG, then the left carotid to LSCA bypass should be constructed to protect the anterior spinal artery. In situations of long-segment aortic endografting, spinal drainage should also be employed. For our specific case

scenario, the LSCA did not need to be covered as there was an adequate proximal landing zone distal to the LSCA. Also, coverage of the LSCA would obstruct the left internal mammary artery, which was used during the coronary bypass procedure 2 weeks prior.

Finally, the timing of TEVAR within 14 days of coronary surgery merits attention. There have been sporadic reports regarding an increased risk of aneurysm rupture in the weeks following an unrelated by major surgery. Most of these reports are anecdotal or retrospective and contain small numbers of patients.[32] A study from the University of Virginia reported 3 of 9 patient (33%) with known AAAs died of aneurysm rupture (avg. size 5.6 cm) between 2 weeks and 6 months following coronary artery bypass surgery.[33] Even though this study contains small numbers of patients, one wouldn't expect 33% of 5.6 cm AAAs to rupture in a 6-month period. Another study from the University of California at San Francisco reports the rupture of 10 asymptomatic AAAs within 36 days (mean 10 days) after a laparotomy for other reasons.[34] It was unclear how many patients had laparotomies with unknown AAAs that did not rupture. However, the rupture of 10 asymptomatic AAAs within 36 days of another surgery seems more than a curiosity. One prospective study from the University of Pittsburg evaluated 33 patients with known AAAs (3.0 to 8.5 cm) who had 45 other unrelated surgeries.[35] The authors concluded no increased risk of AAA rupture, after unrelated surgery, could be identified. However, general anesthesia was used in only 60% of the "other surgeries" and some of the "other surgeries" one might consider as minor operations. Also, 18% of patients in the study had AAAs less than 4.5 cm in diameter. If one were to look at the data and exclude AAAs less than 5 cm in diameter then the aneurysm rupture rate after "other surgery" is 14%. Of the 7 patients who had coronary bypass surgery, there was one AAA rupture (14%) at only 20 days post coronary bypass.

The risk of AAA rupture after coronary surgery is still not conclusively established and the mechanism to explain this phenomenon, if it exists, has not been elucidated. I personally feel there is a relationship between major surgery or a major stress event that may predispose AAAs greater than 5 cm to rupture in the early or midterm post operative period; however, I too have more anecdotes than proof. The aortic wall and the ECM are dynamic structures with continuous collagen/elastin formation and breakdown. Periods of major stress and associated inflammatory mediators in the healing process may weaken the aortic wall ECM and lead to premature aneurysm rupture. Although a biochemical explanation is lacking and conclusive evidence that coronary surgery predisposes to AAA ruptures has not been found, for the specific patient in our case scenario I thought 14 days following coronary surgery was long enough to wait for TAA repair. In general, if a patient has a descending thoracic or abdominal aneurysm with a diameter of 5 cm or greater and undergoes another "major" operation, I would consider repairing their aneurysm promptly.

COMMENTARY

(Joseph S. Coselli, Houston, TX) This chapter reviews the basic etiology, pathology, and common genetic syndromes associated with thoracic aneurysms. The available thoracic endografts from Gore, Medtronic and Cook are presented along with an outline of trial results from Gore and Medtronic. It could be emphasized that the current results for open surgery have substantially improved in recent years. The results of open surgery for open descending thoracic surgery[1], the indication for the on label use of current endovascular devices, carries a mortality and paraplegia rate both below 5%. For thoracoabdominal aortic aneurysm repair, significant strides have also been made, with the use of multiple protective adjuncts, (CSF drainage, Left heart bypass, Hypothermia, etc.) even extent II thoracoabdominal repairs carry a mortality and spinal cord deficit risk of 6% each.[2, 3] Much of the technology around endovascular aortic work represents a transitional phase that is an important transition between historical standards and the day when we will have off the shelf percutaneous devices to address all pathologies; a day we all strive for and a process well represented in this text.

1. Coselli JS. *ATS*. 2004; 77: 1298-1303.
2. Coselli JS. *ATS*. 2007; 83: S862-S864.
3. Coselli JS. *ATS*. 2002; 74: S1881-S1884.

REFERENCES

1. Bickerstall LK, Pairotero PC, Hollier LH, et al. Thoracic aortic aneurysms: A population-based study. *Surg.* 1982; 92: 1103-1108.

2. Vasan RS, Larson MG, Benhamin EJ, Levy D. Echocardiographic reference values for aortic root size. The Framingham Heart Study. *J Am Soc. Echocardiog.* 1995; 8: 793-800.

3. Cronenwett JL and Johnston KW, eds. *Rutherfords Vascular Surgery.* 7th ed. Philadelphia, PA: Saunders-Elsevier; 2010.

4. Andreotti L, Bussotti A, Cammell D, et al. Aortic connective tissue imagery – a biochemical study. *Angiology.* 1985; 36: 872-879.

5. Wolinsky H, Glagov S. A lamellar unit of aortic medial structure and function in mammals. *Civic Research.* 1967; 20: 99-111.

6. Bickerstall LK, Pairolero PC, Hollier LH, et al. Thoracic aortic aneurysms: A population-based study. *Surg.* 1982; 92: 1103-1108.

7. Johansson G, Markstrom U, Swedenborg J. Ruptured thoracic aneurysms: A study of incidence and mortality rates. *J Vasc Surg.* 1995; 21: 985-988.

8. McNamara JJ, Presslet VM. Natural history of arteriosclerotic thoracic aortic aneurysms. *Ann Thorac Surg.* 1978; 26: 468-473.

9. Clouse WD, Hallett JW, Schaff HV, et al. Improved prognosis of thoracic aorta aneurysms: A population-based study. *JAMA.* 1998; 280: 1926-1929.

10. Lumsden AB, Lin PH, Chem C, Parodi JC. Advanced endovascular therapy of aortic disease. Malden, Massachusetts: Blackwell Publishing; 2007.

11. Lee B, Godfrey M, Vitale E, et al. *Linkage of Marfan syndrome and a phenotypically related disorder to two different fibrillin genes.*

12. Pannu H, Tran-Fadulu V, and Milewicz DM. Genetic basis of thoracic aortic aneurysms and aortic dissections. *Amer J Med Genetics Part C.* 2005; 139C: 10-16.

13. Cronenwett JL and Johnston KW, eds. *Rutherfords Vascular.* 7th ed. Philadelphia, PA: Saunders-Elsevier; 2010.

14. Murdoch JL, Walker BA, Hulpern BL, et al. Life expectancy and causes of death in the Marfan syndrome. *N Engl J Med.* 1972; 286: 804-808.

15. Silverman DJ, Burton KL, Gray J, et al. Life expectancy in the Marfan syndrome. *Am J Cardiol.* 1995; 75: 157-160.

16. Superti-Furga A, Steinman B, Byers PH. Type III collagen deficiency. *Lancet.* 1989; 1: 903-904.

17. Superti-Furga A, Guglen E, Gitzelmann R, Steinmann B. Ehlers-Danlos syndrome type IV: A multi-exon deletion in one of the two COL3A1 alleles affecting structure, stability, and processing procollagen. *J Biol Chem.* 1988; 263: 6226-6232.

18. Milewicz D, Guo D, Tran-Fadulu V, et al. Genetic basis of thoracic aortic aneurysms and dissections: Focus on smooth muscle cell contractile dysfunction. *Ann Rev Genomics Hum Genet.* 2008; 9: 283-302.

19. Pepin M, Schwarze U, Superti-Furga A, Byers PH. Clinical and genetic features of Ehlers-Danlos type IV, the vascular type. *N Engl J Med.* 2000; 342: 673-680.

20. Cikrit DF, Miles JH, Silver D. Spontaneous arterial perforation: the Ehlers-Danlos specter. *J Vasc Surg.* 1987; 5: 248-255.

21. Coady MA, Davies RR, Roberts M, et al. Familial patterns of thoracic aortic aneurysms. *Arch of Surg.* 1999; 134: 361-367.

22. Biddinger A, Rocklin M, Coselli J, Milewicz DM. Familial thoracic aortic dilatations and dissections: A case control study. *J Vasc Surg.* 1997; 25: 506-511.

23. Kuang SQ, Guo DC, Prakash SK, et al. Recurrent chromosome 16P13.1 duplications are a risk factor for aortic dissections. 2011 PLOS Gene+ 7 (6): e1002118. Dio: 10,1371/Journal.pgen.1002118.

24. Davies R, Goldstein L, Coady M, et al. Yearly rupture or dissection rates for thoracic aortic aneurysms: Simple prediction based on size. *Ann Thorac Surg.* 2002; 73: 17-28.

25. Dapunt OE, Galla JD, Sadeghi AM, et al. The natural history of thoracic aortic aneurysms. *J Thor Cardiovasc Surg.* 1994; 107: 1323-1332.

26. Perko MJ, Norgaard M, Herzog TM, et al. Unoperated aortic aneurysm: A survey of 170 patients. *Ann Thorac Surg.* 1995; 59 (5): 1204-1209.

27. Stevens SL and Farber MA, eds. *Thoracic Endovascular Aorta.* Knoxville, TN: Tennessee Valley Publishing; 2008.

28. Schermerhorn ML, Giles KA, Hamdan AD, et al. Population-based outcome of open descending thoracic aortic aneurysm repair. *J Vasc Surg.* 2008; 48: 821-827.

29. Coselli JS, LeMaire SA, Conklin LD, Adams GJ. Left heart bypass during descending thoracic aneurysm repair does not reduce the incidence of paraplegia. *Ann Thorac Surg.* 2004; 77 (4): 1298.

30. Makaroun MS, Dillavou ED, Kee ST, et al. Endovascular treatment of thoracic aortic aneurysms: Results of the phase II multicenter trial of the GORE TAG thoracic endoprosthesis. *J Vasc Surg.* 2003; 41: 1-9.

31. Fairman RM, Criado F, Farber M, et al. Pivotal results of the Medtronic vascular Talent thoracic stent graft system: the VALOR trial. *J Vasc Surg.* 2008; 48 (3): 546-554.

32. Ngaage DL, Sulaiman MS, Mavor A, Kaul P. Abdominal aortic aneurysm rupture after coronary artery bypass grafting. *Cardiovasc Surg.* 2003; (11) 3: 237-238.

33. Blackbourne LH, Tribble CG, Langenburg SE, et al. Optimal timing of abdominal aortic aneurysm repair after coronary artery revascularization. *Ann of Surg.* 1994; Vol 219 (6): 693-698.

34. Swanson RJ, Littooy FN, Hunt TK, Stoney RJ. Laparotomy as a precipitating factor in the rupture of intra-abdominal aneurysms. *Arch of Surg.* 1980; 115: 299-304.

35. Durham SJ, Steed DL, Moose HH, et al. Probability of rupture of an abdominal aortic aneurysm after an unrelated operative procedure: A prospective study. *J Vasc Surg.* 1991; 13: 248-252.

CHAPTER 8

Expanding Distal Landing-Zones for Thoracic Endovascular Aortic Aneurysm Repair Using Covered Chimney Grafts

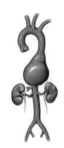

All aneurysms have characteristic nuances and associated risks of repair based upon their location. Similarly, thoracoabdominal aortic aneurysms are problematic as they extend from the thoracic to abdominal cavities. Traditional open repair as required an incision into both the chest and abdomen. The magnitude of the incisions, as well as the need to cross the diaphragm often leads to significant pulmonary complications. Respiratory failure or severe pulmonary complications have been reported in up to 40% of patients[1, 2].

Mortality rates for open thoracoabdominal aortic aneurysm repair may approach 10% even in high volume centers.[3-6] These numbers may actually underestimate the death rate as mortality at one-year postoperative approaches 30%.[6]

Other complications of thoracoabdominal aortic aneurysm repair include renal failure with dialysis required for approximately 10% of patients.[3, 7] One of the most devastating surgical complications is paralysis. Multiple methods have been utilized in an attempt to reduce the risk of paralysis. These methods have included spinal drainage, left heart bypass, retrograde aortic perfusion, hypothermia, and monitoring of sensory/motor evoked potentials. Despite these efforts, the rate of paralysis varies between 5 and 15%.[3, 8-11] Paralysis is certainly related to the length of aorta replaced and the subsequent compromise

of blood flow to the segmental spinal arteries. Coverage or clamping the left subclavian artery will decrease spinal blood flow by occlusion of the anterior spinal artery. In addition, periods of hypotension and/or aortic cross-clamp duration are implicated in the etiology of paralysis.

Endovascular repair and hybrid open/ endovascular rebranching techniques seem to offer a decrease in mortality and major complication rates.[12-17] As discussed in Chapter 5 and 6, the need for available endograft landing zones limits the ability of some patients to receive endograft therapy.

The primary limiting aortic side branch for the distal end of the thoracic aortic endoprosthesis is the celiac artery. In most instances the celiac artery may be sacrificed or covered by the endograft without the harmful sequelae of visceral ischemia.[18, 19] This requires careful preoperative assessment of collateral blood flow between the superior mesenteric artery and the celiac artery via the gastro-duodenal artery. However, this major collateral pathway is not complete in all patients and the consequences of celiac artery occlusion may be immediate hepatic/intestinal infarction or a more indolent presentation of ischemia days post operatively if relative hypotension or metabolic demands interfere with the balance of collateral flow. Other patients who should not undergo celiac

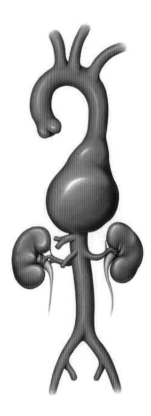

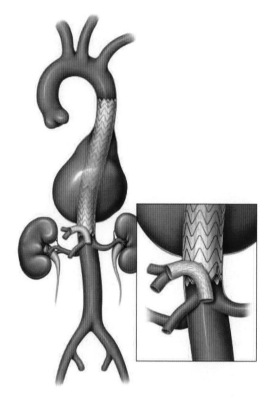

Figure 8-1 Illustration of 10 centimeter aneurysm with relation to celiac artery.

Figure 8-2 Illustration of repaired aneurysm with chimney graft in celiac artery. Relationship of celiac graft to main body of graft (inset).

occlusion are those with underlying liver disease, previous pancreatic surgery, or a history of portal vein thrombosis. The below case scenario details the use of a covered chimney graft to preserve celiac artery blood flow during thoracic endovascular aneurysm repair.

CASE SCENARIO:
Expanding Distal Thoracic Aortic Landing-Zones

A 66-year-old man presented to the cardiology service with exacerbation of congestive heart failure. Comorbidities included cardiomyopathy (ejection fracture 25 percent), chronic obstructive pulmonary disease requiring chronic home-oxy-

gen therapy, diabetes, multiple previous coronary artery stents, and morbid obesity. Cardiac catheterization suggested a thoracic aortic aneurysm extending below the diaphragm. Subsequent computerized tomography demonstrated a thoracoabdominal aortic aneurysm with a maximum diameter of 10 cm and extending within 1 cm of the celiac artery. The patient was not a candidate for open surgical therapy primarily because of poor baseline pulmonary function and obesity. Endograft therapy with celiac artery preservation was planned. Figure 8-1 illustrates the extent of the aneurysm.

Under general anesthesia, the right and left femoral arteries were exposed by cutdown. Using standard endovascular technique 0.035 inch thoracic graft was then deployed so that the distal end of the endograft extended approximately 2 cm below the native celiac artery ostia. The distal end of the celiac graft extended just below the thoracic graft as seen in figure 8-2. Note: Chimney grafts do not take a true 90 degree course, but often spiral along the main graft within the aorta. The procedure was completed by placing two additional telescoping thoracic endografts more proximally; sizes 37 mm by 10 cm and size 40 mm by 10 cm, respectively. The larger diameter grafts are always placed inside the smaller grafts. The patient remains in his baseline state of poor health two years post procedure. Computerized tomographic angiogram demonstrates no endoleak and a patent chimney graft with contrast visualized in the celiac artery, figure 8-3. The axial cut demonstrates the relationship of the chimney to the main grafts, figure 8-4.

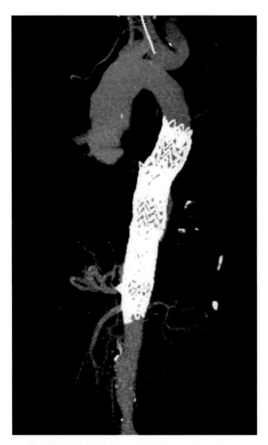

Figure 8-3 Computerized tomographic angiogram. Note celiac artery chimney graft extending below main body graft. Note flow in celiac and splenic arteries.

guidewire was placed in the ascending aorta. A 24-Fr sheath was positioned in the upper abdominal aorta over the stiff guidewire. Because of the patient's obesity, the 24-Fr sheath was placed through a separate stab incision, this allowed for less angulation as the sheath entered the femoral artery. Similarly, a 12-Fr sheath was placed in the contralateral femoral artery. Using the 12-Fr sheath as access, the celiac artery was cannulated and an 8 mm by 5 cm Viabahn covered chimney graft was positioned in the celiac artery. Simultaneously, via the 24-Fr sheath, a TAG endoprosthesis size 31 mm by 10 cm was positioned in the aorta. The celiac artery stent graft was deployed first leaving approximately 1.5 cm of graft in the celiac artery and 3.5 cm directed distally into the aorta. The

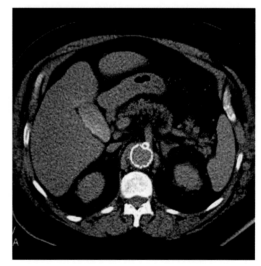

Figure 8-4 Axial cut of computerized tomogram demonstrating relationship of chimney to main graft.

REFERENCES

1. Eagle J, Soli HJ, Miller III CC, et al. The Impact of Diaphragm Management on Prolonged Ventilator Support After Thoracoabdominal Aortic Repair. *Journal of Vascular Surgery.* 1999; 29: 150-156.

2. Rectenwald JE, Huber TS, Martin TD, et al. Functional Outcome After Thoracoabdominal Aortic Aneurysm Repair. *Journal of Vascular Surgery.* 2002; 35: 640-647.

3. Svensson LG, Crawford ES, Hess KR et al. Experience With 1509 Patients Undergoing Thoracoabdominal Aortic Operations. *Journal of Vascular Surgery.* 1993; 17: 357-368.

4. Derrow AE, Seeger JM, Dame DA, et al. The Outcome in the United States After Thoracoabdominal Aortic Aneurysm Repairs, Renal Artery Bypass, and Mesentric Revascularisation. *Journal of Vascular Surgery.* 2001; 34: 54-61.

5. Cowan JA, Dimick JB, Jenke PK, et al. Surgical Treatment of Intact Thoracoabdominal Aortic Aneurysms in the United States: Hospital and Surgeon Volume-Related Outcomes. *Journal of Vascular Surgery.* 2003; 37: 1169-1174.

6. Riberg DA, McGory ML, Zingmond DS, et al. Thirty-Day Mortality Statistics Underestimate the Risk of Repair of Thoracoabdominal Aortic Aneurysms Repair: A Statewide Experience. *Journal of Vascular Surgery.* 2006; 43: 217-222.

7. Hassoun HT, Miller III CC, Huynh TT, et al. Cold Visceral Perfusion Improves Early Survival in Patients with Acute Renal Failure After Thoracoabdominal Aortic Aneurysm Repair. *Journal of Vascular Surgery.* 2004; 506-512.

8. Coselli JS, Conklin LD, LeMaire SA. Thoracoabdominal Aortic Aneurysm Repair: Review and Update on Current Strategies. *Annals of Thoracic Surgery.* 2002; 74: 51881-51884.

9. Zvara DA. Thoracoadominal Aortic Aneurysm Surgery and the Risk of Paraplegia: Contemporary Practice and Future Directions. *Journal of Extracorporeal Technology.* 2002; 34: 11-17.

10. Safi HJ, Estrera AL, Miller CC, et al. Evolution of Risk for Neurologic Deficit After Descending and Thoracoabdominal Aortic Repair. *Annals of Thoracic Surgery.* 2005; 80: 2173-2179.

11. Svensson LG. Paralysis After Aortic Surgery: In Search of Lost Cord Function. *Surgeon.* 2005; 3: 396-405.

12. Lee AW, Brown MP, Martin TD, et al. Early Results After Staged Hybrid Repair of Thoracoabdominal Aortic Aneurysms. *Journal of American College of Surgeons.* 2007; 205; 420-431.

13. Hughs CG, Nienaber JJ, Bush EL, et al. Use of Custom Dacron Branch Grafts for "Hybrid" Aortic Debranching During Endovascular Repair of Thoracic and Thoracoabdominal Aortic Aneurysms. *Journal of Thoracic and Cardiovascular Surgery.* 2008; 136: 21-28.

14. Diethrich EB, Ramaiah VG, Kpodonu J, Rodriguez-Lopez JA. *Endovascular and Hybrid Management of the Thoracic Aorta.* Hoboken, NJ: Wiley-Blackwell Publishing; 2008.

15. Fairman RA, Criado F, Farber M, et al. Pivotal Results of the Medtronic Vascular talent Thoracic Stent Graft System: The VALOR Trial. *Journal of Vascular Surgery.* 2008; 48: 546-554.

16. Makaroun MS, Dillavou ED, Kes ST, et al. Endovascular Treatment of Thoracic Aortic Aneurysms: Results of the Phase II Multicenter Trial of the Gore TAG Thoracic Endoprosthesis. *Journal of Vascular Surgery.* 2005; 41: 1-9.

17. Greenberg RK, O'Neil S, Walker E, et al. Endovascular Repair of Thoracic Aortic Lesions with the Zenith Tx1 and Tx2 Thoracic Grafts (Intermediate-Term Results). *Journal of Vascular Surgery.* 2005; 41: 589-596.

18. Vaddineni S, Taylor S, Patterson W, et al. Outcome After Celiac Artery Coverage During Endovascular Thoracic Aortic Aneurysm Repair: Preliminary Results. *Journal of Vascular Surgery.* 2007; Volume 45 (3): 467-471.

19. Leon LR, Mills JL, Jordan W, et al. The Risks of Celiac Artery Coverage During Endoluminal Repair of Thoracic and Thoracoabdominal Aortic Aneurysms. *Vascular and Endovascular Surgery.* 2009; 43 (1): 51-60.

CHAPTER 9

Re-operative Repair of a 9 Centimeter Thoracoabdominal Aortic Aneurysm, Five Years after an Elephant-Trunk Procedure with 11- and 16-Year Follow-up

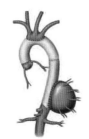

Surgical repair of aneurysms involving the transverse and descending aorta have been associated with an overall mortality of 4.4 – 31%.[1-4] The elephant trunk technique described by Borst in 1983 allowed for a two-stage repair of extensive aneurysms with a decrease in operative mortality.[5] Reports from large centers describe a 2-12% operative mortality for stage-one elephant trunk and a 3.9 – 9.6% mortality for the second stage.[6-8] However, a subset of patients have a descending thoracic aortic aneurysm that involves the renomesenteric vessels of the abdominal aorta. Other patients have an extensive thoracoabdominal aneurysm (TAAA) that also involves the ascending aorta. Little is published regarding the open mortality of patients with total aortic aneurysm. The elective repair of pure thoracoabdominal aortic aneurysm (left subclavian to distal) have an elective operative mortality of 22% in The United States. The operative mortality for a ruptured TAAA is 54%.[9]

In addition to mortality concerns, the risk of paralysis is significant and preserving spinal cord perfusion is critical in both case planning and technique. The anterior spinal artery arises from the left subclavian artery superiorly. Aortic clamping proximal to the left subclavian artery or occluding the left subclavian artery will increase the risk of paralysis. The risk is related to the length of time of cross-clamping and to the extent of aorta

replaced. If the aneurysm extends through the level of the renomesenteric arteries, important intercostal arteries will be involved. The artery radicularis magnus, which contributes to the anterior spinal artery from below, originates between T4 and T12 in 75% of the population.[10] Often numerous intercostal arteries are occluded by thrombus within the aneurysm sac or are relatively small and may be "unimportant." Determining which intercostal arteries are "important" for spinal cord protection is the subject of much debate. The intraoperative use of motor evoked potentials (MEPs) is helpful in determining which intercostal arteries should be re-implanted. Clearly, all large intercostal artery pairs, especially those with minimal back-bleeding, should be reattached and if possible all patent intercostal arteries between T8 and L1 should be preserved.

The following case presentation is a late complicating occurring after the successful repair of a thoracoabdominal aortic aneurysm with re-implantation of five intercostal artery pairs during the second stage of an elephant trunk procedure.

CASE SCENARIO:
Thoracoabdominal Aortic Aneurysm

The patient is a 63-year-old, white woman who had a successful two-stage elephant trunk procedure in

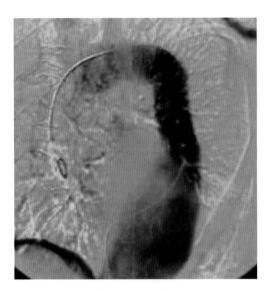

Figure 9-1 Preoperative aortogram of 9 cm thoracoabdominal aortic aneurysm, proximal aspect.

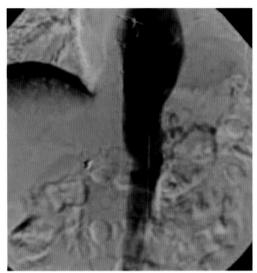

Figure 9-2 Preoperative aortogram of 9 cm thoracoabdominal aortic aneurysm, distal aspect.

1995. The operative procedure at that time involved replacing the ascending aorta and re-implanting the cerebral head vessels as an island patch to repair the transverse arch aneurysm. A distal elephant trunk anastomosis was constructed. The aortic valve and coronary arteries were without significant pathology. The second stage consisted of a thoracoabdominal incision with a standard graft-to-trunk anastomosis proximally and re-implantation of five pairs of intercostal arteries (T8 through T12) as a long patch graft. The distal graft had a beveled anastomosis to replace excised aneurysmal tissue to the level of the mesenteric arteries. Postoperatively from that procedure in 1995, the patient had no neurologic deficits.

Five years later, the patient presented to the emergency department with sudden onset of severe upper back pain. Computerized tomography demonstrated a 9 cm aneurysm of the distal thoracic/proximal abdominal aorta. An anastomotic aneurysm of the intercostal artery patch was postulated. The patient remained hemodynamically stable, although active hemorrhage could not be completely excluded. Two views of the patient's preoperative aortogram are seen in figures 9-1 and 9-2.

In the operating room, the patient was positioned in the oblique right lateral decubitus position. A re-operative thoracoabdominal incision was performed through approximately the sixth rib interspace and into the abdomen. The pertinent operative findings were a 9 cm aneurysm of the aortic tissue containing the five pairs of re-implanted intercostal arteries. Figure 9-3 illustrates the intraoperative findings. No back-bleeding was encountered from the intercostal arteries and in consideration of this reoperative status and the time interval for collateral artery development since the first surgery, I chose not to re-implant these intercostal arteries. Indeed, the reoperative nature of this procedure added to the case complexity and the surgery was complicated by an avulsion injury to the spleen, necessitating splenectomy.

At the time of the original operation in 1995, the aortic valve and root were not replaced. Some concern is justified for the potential development of a sinus of Valsalva aneurysm. However, at 16 years post procedure, that has not happened. At this time, the patient has normal neurologic and renal function. She is a 16-year survivor from her elephant trunk procedure and an 11-year survivor from her reoperative thoracoabdominal aortic aneurysm surgery. Figure 9-4 is the most recent CT scan from 2010, showing again successful repair with no aneurysmal development of the aorta. Clearly the reimplantation of intercostal arteries as a "patch" has reduced the incidence of paralysis. However, these patients should be in a surveillance system, just as endograft patients in order to asses for the development of paraanastomotic aneurysms.

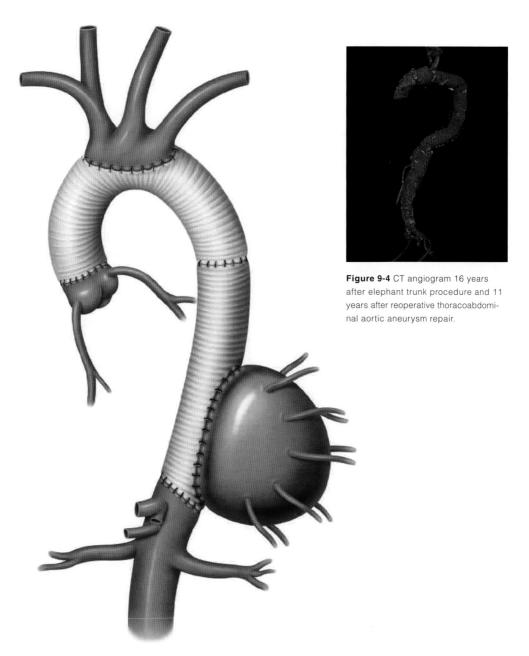

Figure 9-4 CT angiogram 16 years after elephant trunk procedure and 11 years after reoperative thoracoabdominal aortic aneurysm repair.

Figure 9-3 Illustration of aneurysm at attachment of intercostal arteries at prior elephant trunk procedure.

COMMENTARY

(Hazim J. Safi, Houston, TX) The chapter opens with an excellent review of the rationale for the elephant trunk procedure as a report regarding repair of extensive aortic aneurysms: ascending, arch and thoracoabdominal aortic segments. There are reports regarding the use of deep hypothermia and circulatory arrest for patients with extensive aortic aneurysm. We do not prefer that method due to troublesome intraoperative coagulopathy.

In the introduction, there is a good review of spinal cord blood supply and anatomy. Our group also recognizes the importance of the left subclavian artery as a contributor to the spinal cord blood supply via the left vertebral artery. Clamp placement proximal to the left subclavian artery adversely affects spinal blood supply. As we discovered in thoracic endografting, coverage of the origin of the left subclavian artery without prior revascularization increases the risk of stroke[1] and may increase risk of spinal paralysis.[2] Currently, we guide our reattachment of intercostals arteries #8-12 by neuromonitoring of the spinal cord. In our most recent data, 3% of patients required the attachment of intercostals arteries as determined by changes in somatosensory or motor evoked potentials or both.

Following this brief introduction, the case of redo thoracoabdominal aortic aneurysm with an intercostal patch was described succinctly. A 63-year old woman had a successful repair of a proximal aortic aneurysm 16 years ago. She returned five years later with an aneurysm of the intercostal artery patch. Given the proximity of the patch aneurysm to the celiac artery, it is likely that the patient was not a suitable candidate for the endovascular repair. The intraoperative decision was made to forego intercostal artery reimplantation with a successful result. In our practice, we would have used a neuromonitoring-guided approach. If no changes on somatosensory or motor evoked potentials, we would have proceeded with the ligation of intercostal arteries.[3] Otherwise, we would reimplant the intercostal arteries via a side-to-side loop graft attached to the main body aortic graft.

The follow-up of the patient was excellent. I was impressed with the clean line drawings and illustrations without clutter. That is credit to the cooperative efforts between the surgeon and the illustrator. This chapter and the book as a whole, is a valuable asset to the practicing surgeon who is interested in dealing with the complex pathology of the aorta. The author is to be congratulated in producing such an excellent book.

---

1. Chung J, Kasirajan K, Veeraswamy RK, et al. Left subclavian coverage during thoracic endovascular aortic repair and risk of perioperative stroke or death. *J Vasc Surg*. 2011; 54: 979-84.
2. Holt PJ, Johnson C, Hinchliffe RJ, et al. Outcomes of the endovascular management of aortic arch aneurysm: implications for management of the left subclavian artery. *J Vasc Surg*. 2010; 51: 1329-38.
3. Estera AL, Sheinbaum R, Miller CC, 3rd, Harrison R, Safi HJ. Neuromonitor-guided repair of thoracoabdominal aortic aneurysms. *J Thorac Cardiovasc Surg*. 2010; 140: S131-5; discussion S42-S46.

REFERENCES

1. Cooley DA, Golmon, Frazier OH. Single-clamp technique for aneurysm of the descending thoracic aorta: Report on 132 consecutive cases. *Eur J Cardiothoracic Surg.* 2000; 18 (2): 162-167.

2. Estrera Al, Miller III CC, Chen EP, et al. Descending thoracic aortic aneurysm repair: 12-year experience using distal aortic perfusion and cerebrospinal fluid drainage. *Ann Thorac Surg.* 2005; 80 (4): 1290.

3. Stone, OH, Brewster DC, Kwolek CJ, et al. Stent-graft versus open surgical repair of the thoracic aorta: midterm results. *J. Vasc Surg.* 2006; 44 (6): 1188.

4. Verdant A, Crossett R, et al. Aneurysms of the descending thoracic aorta: Three hundred sixty-six cases resected without paraplegia. *J. Vasc Surg.* 1995; 21(3): 385.

5. Borst H G, Walterbusch G, Schaps D. Extensive aortic replacement using "elephant trunk" prosthesis. *Thoracic Cardiovasc Surg.* 1983; 31 (1): 37-40.

6. Safi HJ, Miller III CC, Estrera AL, et al. Optimization of aortic arch replacement: Two-stage approach. *Ann Thorac Surg.* 2007; 87 (2): S 815-818.

7. LeMaire SA, Carter SA, Coselli JS. The elephant trunk technique for staged repair of the entire thoracic aorta. *Ann Thorac Surg.* 2006; 81 (5): 1561-1569.

8. Svensson LG, Kim KH, Blackstone EH, et al. Elephant trunk procedure: Newer indications and uses. *Ann Thorac Surg.* 2004; 781 (1): 109-116.

9. Cronenwett JL, Johnston KW, eds. *Rutherford's Vascular Surgery.* 7th ed. Philadelphia, PA: Elsevier Saunders; 2010.

10. Coselli JS, Lemaire SA. Descending and thoracoabdominal aortic aneurysm. In: L H Cohn (Ed), Cardiac Surgery in the Adult, 3rd Edition. McGraw-Hill, New York, 2008: 1277-1289.

CHAPTER 10

Management Strategies for Blunt Trauma to the Thoracic Aorta

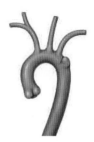

Blunt aortic injury is a leading cause of death from blunt force trauma.[1-3] The often cited 1958 report from the Armed Forces Institute of Pathology concluded that 75-80% of all patients with blunt aortic injury die at the scene of the accident.[4] Of the patients arriving alive at the hospital, 50% will die in the following week. The lethality of this injury led to intense efforts to rapidly diagnose and treat this ominous condition. Over the last 30 years, the scientific literature has been replete with controversy regarding diagnostic modalities, treatment techniques, and the timing of therapy.[5-12] Lack of universal consensus was fueled by the

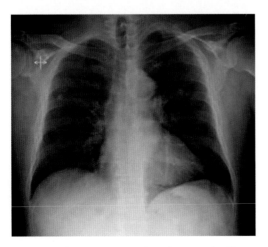

Figure 10-1 Chest roentogram of aortic transection. Note double-density at aortic knob.

overall poor prognosis of the injury and the inability of any treatment strategy to demonstrate conclusive superiority.

Currently, interest has shifted to minimally invasive endovascular management of blunt aortic injury. Over 400 small-series reports demonstrate virtually no instance of paralysis with endovascular aortic repair.[13-17] However, this, too, has generated more questions and controversy as no endovascular device meets the United States Food and Drug Administration approval for this application. Additionally, concerns regarding aortic growth and the long-term durability of endovascular devices in the relatively young trauma patient population are justified. Even the sacred tenant of immediate aortic repair is under scrutiny as the true incidence of aortic rupture after arrival to the hospital may be less than previously believed.[18-25] A subset of patients with aortic injury may be better served with "delayed" endovascular or even "delayed" open-repair.[26-36]

The following case scenario and discussion will address these issues.

CASE SCENARIO:
Aortic Injury

The patient is a 54-year-old man who presented to his family physician with a persistent cough. Chest

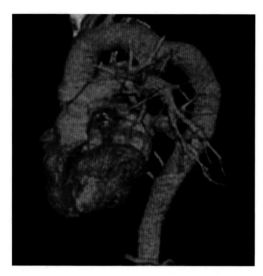

Figure 10-2 Computerized tomographic scan of chronic traumatic thoracic aortic transection.

x-ray demonstrated a widened mediastinum, figure 10-1. Pertinent past medical history included a three week hospitalization at another facility following a high speed motor vehicle accident over two years previously. The patient had sustained a right femoral fracture, facial fractures, and a right hand trauma during that accident. Subsequent computerized tomography, figure 10-2, and the artist's illustration indicate a traumatic aortic

transection distal to the left subclavian artery with a current diameter of the aorta in this area at 7 cm, figure 10-3.

Under general anesthesia, the patient's common femoral artery was identified by cutdown. A soft-tip 0.035 inch guide wire was advanced into the ascending aorta under fluoroscopic visualization. The soft wire was exchanged through a protective guide catheter for a 0.035 inch stiff wire. After systemic heparinization, a 22-Fr sheath was advanced over the stiff guide wire. Using a buddy wire technique, a pigtail marking catheter was positioned in the ascending aorta through the same femoral sheath. A subsequent aortogram with 60 degree left anterior oblique angulation demonstrates the aortic transection, figure 10-4. A thoracic endograft size 34 mm by 15 cm was deployed to exclude the area of transection. A tri-lobed balloon was used to fully appose the graft to the aortic wall. The tri-lobed balloon allows for 3-point contact to expand the endograft and still permit aortic blood flow to pass through the balloon. A completely occlusive balloon high in the aortic arch would be prone to "bounce" distally during systolic with potential intimal disruption or endograft migration. The aortogram following graft deployment demonstrates exclusion of the

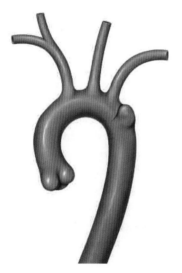

Figure 10-3 Illustration of thoracic aortic transection.

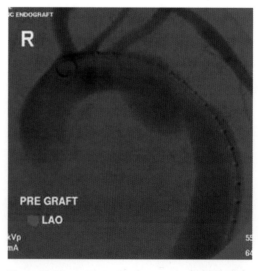

Figure 10-4 Intraoperative aortogram prior to endograft placement.

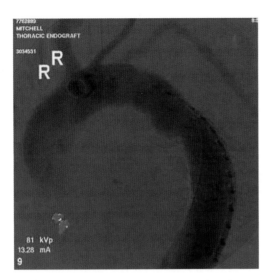

Figure 10-5 Intraoperative aortogram post-endograft placement.

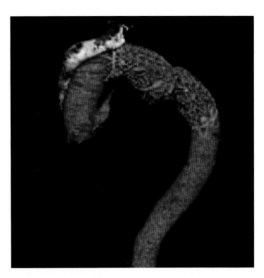

Figure 10-6 Computerized tomographic angiogram post-endograft.

transection and no evidence of endoleak, figure 10-5. This repair has remained durable for four years without graft migration, endoleak, or proximal graft collapse, figure 10-6.

CASE DISCUSSION:
Blunt Aortic Injury

The above patient illustrates a number of issues regarding blunt aortic injury. First, the patient was involved in a motor vehicle accident. This mechanism of injury accounts for 90% of all cases of blunt aortic trauma. Secondly, the milder degree of this patient's aortic disruption probably accounted for his ability to survive greater than two years from the time of his accident. Blunt aortic injury is a spectrum of injury extending from intimal hemorrhage, intimal laceration, medial laceration, to complete aortic laceration.[4] Although only speculation, if this patient initially sustained a low level intimal or medial laceration, there would be minimal or no mediastinal widening on initial chest x-ray. This could account for his aortic injury being undiagnosed years prior at the time of his accident. As this patient now has aortic enlargement to 7 cm, the risk of rupture is substantial and prompt, although not emergency

repair is recommended. Patients such as this, presenting years after the original aortic injury, have prompted some surgeons to consider delayed aortic repair at the time of initial presentation if the injury disruption appears small and there are significant other associated injuries.[18-20, 23]

In the case of an acutely injured patient with multiple organ trauma, if spiral CT angiography demonstrated a small medial laceration without significant aortic enlargement, consideration may be given to delayed aortic repair. Strict blood pressure control to avoid hypertension is necessary during this period of observation. Once the patient is stabilized from associated injuries, the aortic injury may be addressed. Unfortunately, once the surgeon is aware that an aortic injury exists, distinguishing a "small" from a "large" injury is difficult in a litiginous society.

For our patient in this discussion presenting years after aortic injury, open surgery is certainly an appealing option. Open surgery requires a thoracotomy with a hand-sutured interposition graft to repair the aorta. The three main variations of the open technique include: clamp and sew, shunting, and left-heart bypass. Clamp and sew is essentially only that. The aorta is clamped proximally and distally to the injury, the injured aorta is resected and an interposition graft is sutured to reestablish aortic continuity. The clamp and sew technique has a time-dependent relationship with paralysis. If the aortic continuity is not reestablished in 30 minutes, the risk of paralysis increases.[39] Although a number of studies suggest the risk of paralysis with the clamp and sew method is unacceptably high, some surgeons have had excellent results with this technique.[8] The principle advantage to the clamp and sew technique is that it does not require systemic heparinization; this is an important consideration in the trauma patient with multiple concomitant injuries or an intracranial hemorrhage.

Brand	Smallest Diameter (mm)
Medtronic Talent	22
Gore TAG	26
Zenith	28

Figure 10-7 Commercially available thoracic endografts in the United States with smallest diameters (mm) as of August 2011.

The shunting technique primarily involves the use of the Gott shunt. The Gott shunt is a plastic tube of approximately 9 mm in diameter. One end of the shunt is generally inserted into the ascending aorta using purse-string sutures. The other end is inserted into the distal thoracic aorta or femoral artery. This allows perfusion of the distal aorta and allows for unloading left ventricular wall stress during aortic cross clamping. This technique can be performed with a minimal amount of heparin and paralysis rates have been very low in some series.[10] The Gott shunt has not gained widespread acceptance as the shunt can be cumbersome. In addition, as the flow in the shunt is passive, distal perfusion pressure cannot be as well controlled as in left-heart bypass.

Left-heart bypass has become one of the most used techniques for open aortic repair. Left-heart bypass involves placing a cannula in the left atrial appendage and another in the distal aorta or common femoral artery with a centrifugal pump

in between. This has the advantage of perfusing the distal aorta, and thus the spinal cord with blood under relatively controlled flow and pressure. In addition, left-heart bypass relieves left ventricular strain during cross-clamping. By maintaining distal aortic perfusion and relieving left ventricular strain, longer cross clamp times can be achieved with minimal increase in paralysis. Critics of left heart bypass are concerned about potential deleterious effects of systemic heparinization in the trauma patient. Except in cases of intracranial hemorrhage, I believe that those fears are overstated. With the current use of heparin-bonded tubing and centrifugal pumps, the need for heparin is minimal. Despite the advances of left-heart bypass with a centrifugal pump, the paralysis risk of acute aortic repair is still 3% in large series.[3]

Finally, the risk of paralysis is very different for the open repair of an acute versus a chronic aortic transection. Patients presenting years after their original aortic injury have undergone open-repair with minimal risk of paralysis.[32] The reasons for this are not fully understood but speculation extends from less labile blood pressure than would be found in those patients in the chronic trauma phase, to selection of more experienced high volume aortic surgery centers for elective repair of chronic transections.

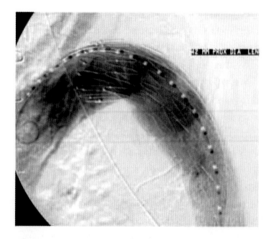

Figure 10-8 "Bird-Beaking". Note lower edge of endograft is not apposed to inner curve of acutely angled aorta. Courtesy of Cook Medical.

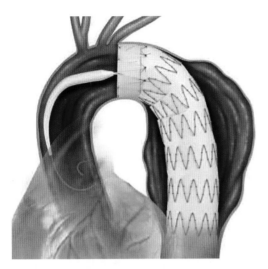

Figure 10-9 Model of Proform TX-2 endograft in aorta to eliminate bird-beaking. Courtesy of Cook Medical.

The application of endografts to treat aortic transections seems intuitive. The procedure is minimally invasive and avoids a thoracotomy incision. The technique can be performed with minimal or no heparin. Most importantly, multiple small series have demonstrated virtually no instances of paralysis.[13-16] Endografting for traumatic aortic transections has no doubt been life-saving for many patients. However, there are a number of issues to consider.

At this time, there are no thoracic endografts approved by the United States Food and Drug Administration for the treatment of aortic transections. Currently, studies are underway to expand the indications of thoracic endografts to include aortic trauma. But for now, both the surgeon and the patient's family should be aware that a widely-accepted, albeit "unapproved" procedure, is being performed for a critically ill patient.

Anatomic considerations make endograft repair of the aortic transection problematic. The average age of the trauma population is relatively young at 34 years.[3] Young patients tend to have a smaller aortic diameter and a more acutely angled aortic arch. The acute angle may impede full expansion of the endograft against the inner curvature of the aorta. This can result in the so-called "bird-beak" effect, figure 10-8. Bird-beaking can contribute to endoleak, graft migration, and catastrophic graft collapse. Figure 10-9 demonstrates the Proform TX-2 thoracic endograft (Cook Medical Inc, Bloomington, IN). The flexible proximal end of this device may minimize or eliminate bird-beaking. Another endograft, the C-TAG (W. L. Gore and Assoc., Flagstaff, AZ) may be beneficial in aortic transections. However, the C-TAG will not be released for general use until late 2011.

In addition to aortic arch angulation, the small aortic diameter in many trauma patients is an obstacle to endografting. One study found the mean aortic diameter in patients with traumatic aortic transections was 19.3 mm.[40] Commercially available endografts with the smallest sizes (diameter) manufactured are listed in figure 10-7. However, with aortas smaller than 19 mm, even the smallest thoracic endografts may be "oversized" and lead to graft enfolding and collapse. The conformable-TAG (C-TAG), which is in clinical trials, has not been approved by the FDA at this time. The smallest C-TAG has a diameter of 21 mm and can land in an aorta with a diameter of 16 mm.

One alternative to managing transections in the small thoracic aorta has been the use of abdominal aortic endograft extension cuffs.[14] These are readily available as off-the-shelf components. As they were originally designed for the abdominal aorta, they are manufactured in smaller diameters and therefore be more likely to match the small diameters of a thoracic aorta in a young trauma patient. Unfortunately, the delivery catheters for the abdominal endografts are relatively short. In taller patients, they may not be able to reach the thoracic arch.

Even with the ability of some small thoracic endografts or abdominal extension grafts to treat thoracic aortic transections, two other potential problems remain. First, the aorta is known to grow and expand as the patient ages. The 20-year stability of an endograft in a young trauma patient whose native aorta will enlarge over time is unknown. Secondly, the 20-year structural durability of the endograft material itself is also unknown. However, when considering the lethality of aortic trauma and the risk of paralysis associated with open surgery in the acute setting, endovascular success for even 10 years is an attractive option.[41] Additionally, endovascular repair in the acute setting does not preclude open surgical repair years later in a more elective situation.

For the patient in our case scenario, he was 54 years of age with a mature "uncoiled" aorta, figure 10-2. An endograft in the patient would not be prone to bird-beaking as there was no acute arch angulation. Also, the mature aorta was unlikely to grow to a significant degree in this patient's lifetime. Although open surgical repair for a chronic transection is certainly an appealing alternative, the patient strongly preferred the endovascular approach. The size 34 mm endograft was appropriately sized and has remained durable without migration, endoleak or collapse at four years post procedure.

In summary, blunt aortic injury is essentially a disease of modern society as over 90% of cases are attributed to automobile or motorcycle accidents.[3] Similarly, one can see modern surgery's evolution in the diagnosing and management of this injury over a relatively short time frame of 30-40 years. Diagnosis has evolved from autopsy and chest x-ray to aortogram and spiral CT angiography. Treatment has included "clamp and sew", partial bypass or shunt techniques, and now endovascular repair. Timing of repair depends upon associated injuries and the "degree" of aortic injury. Blunt aortic trauma is still controversial in many respects. Pitfalls in understanding the evolution of aortic injury management are the assumption that all evolution is continually forward and the tendency to believe that we, as surgeons, are practicing in the final states of that evolutionary process. Undoubtedly, new advances will emerge. Although protocols and algorithms have their place, the best management of blunt aortic injury must be determined on a case by case basis. Ultimately, that will require the application of the most elusive of qualities: surgical experience and surgical judgment.

COMMENTARY

(Baron L. Hamman, Dallas, TX) Mere discovery of the angiographic abnormality is not an independent indication for operation although it would push the surgeon toward therapy in the absence of other more pressing illness and in the setting of anticipated viable longevity. Though the diagnosis was initially missed, the case illustrates the value of delayed treatment. In the setting of complex multi-trauma patients – particularly those with perfusion and edema dependent injury (closed brain injury, liver laceration, pulmonary contusion are the most commonly concomitantly diagnosed) – delay may offer a life saving window in which the coagulation system can recover or damage to an organ can "ebb and flow" thus allowing the arterial operation a new window for likely successful intervention. Timing is the critical element for establishing the risk/benefit equation; further the equation must be specific to patient and doctor expectations.

The Thoracic Aortic Endovascular Repair (TEVAR) technique is gaining wide acceptance though the caveats of age and growth are addressed in the case discussion. The lesser morbidity associated with percutaneous covered stent deployment in the setting of descending aortic dissections (newly diagnosed) and the "off label" or "study" use of TEVAR in traumatic transection have led some leading centers to perform this procedure preferentially.

The open techniques are addressed though they are principally of a historical or comparison importance. Be aware that many recently trained surgeons will have only limited experience with the open techniques and may not be comfortable (or adept) with the open thoracotomy method of repair.

COMMENTARY

(Kenneth L. Mattox, Houston, TX) This chapter uses a clinical case study to underscore advances that have occurred in the diagnosis and management of blunt aortic trauma. However, like much of the recent literature on the subject of blunt aortic trauma, the chapter is limited, in that it focuses entirely on the proximal descending thoracic aorta. Up to 30% of thoracic aortic injuries occur in other locations. Currently, these other locations (aortic root, ascending aortic, or aortic arch/innominate artery) are approached completely different from those in the descending thoracic aorta, for both open and endovascular approaches.[2, 4]

The knowledge base on understanding, diagnosing, and managing aortic trauma has evolved over the past 50 years, with each decade focusing on a different debate. The early debates on causes of death in these patients were replaced by controversies on screening and diagnosis techniques. Subsequently, the use of afterload reduction allowed for purposeful delay in thoracic aortic injury management, especially in patients with multisystem injury to the brain, lungs, and abdomen.[2, 3] It is logical that endovascular approaches for many patients with injury to the proximal descending thoracic aortic should be applied and that multicenter series should be reported.[1]

In reported comparative series, the results of endovascular management of a descending thoracic aortic repair with an endograft are significantly better than for traditional open approaches. However, the case mix is not the same between these groups. Emerging concerns are raised in four areas: (1) endograft –aortic diameter mismatch resulting in enfolding, (2) covering of aortic branch vessels, (3) damage to the introducer entry site, and (4) Long-term outcomes in patients whose aortas continue to dilate over time. One additional concern is that with time, the accumulated experience and expertise needed to perform cases that require immediate or delayed open management is in danger of being lost.

Finally, it is imperative endograft insertion not be the management choice for patients with "trivial, minimal, or no injury" to the aortic wall. It is quite possible that with the singular use of CT as a diagnostic methodology, a significant percentage (potentially up to 30%) of the thoracic endografts deployed for blunt thoracic aortic trauma are inserted in aortas with minimal intimal injury that required no therapy.

---

1. Demetriades D, Velmahos GC, Scalea TM, et al. Blunt traumatic aortic injuries: Early or delayed repair – Results of an American Association for the Surgery of trauma perspective study. *J Trauma.* 2009; 66: 967-973.
2. Mattox KL, Red River Anthology. *J Trauma.* 1997; March 42 (3): 353-368.
3. Mattox KL, Wall MJ Jr., Wagner RB, Faber PF, eds. *Historical Review of Blunt Injury to the Thoracic Aorta.* Chapter in Chest Surgery Clinics of North America. Philadelphia, PA: WB Saunders Co; February 2000.
4. Teixeira, PGR, Inaba K, Barmparas G, et al. Blunt Thoracic Aortic Injuries: An Autopsy Study. *J Trauma.* 2011; 70: 197-202.

AUTHOR'S RESPONSE

I find it interesting that both Drs. Hamman (directly) and Mattox (indirectly) chose to express their concerns that the skills necessary to perform complex "open" surgery may be diminishing as vascular surgery training has become dominated by endovascular procedures. I share their concerns. Recently, in a report of graduating vascular fellows from U.S. training programs, the average graduate performed 0.5 open renal artery bypass procedures during their training. Another interpretation of that data is that one-half of the physicians being trained as vascular surgeon specialists have never performed the operation. I recognize that renal artery bypass may be an extreme example as currently the procedure is seldom needed. But, I am certain that this trend extends to some degree for other "open" operations within the spectrum of vascular surgery, such as the open repair of ruptured abdominal aortic aneurysms. Indeed, some skills are in danger of being lost.

REFERENCES

1. Pasaro E, Pace WB. Traumatic rupture of the aorta. *Surgery.* 1959; 46: 787.
2. Smith RS, Chang FC. Traumatic rupture of the aorta: Still a lethal injury. *Am J Surg.* 1986; 152: 660.
3. Fabian TC, Richardson JD, Croce MA, et al. Prospective study of blunt aortic injury: Multicenter Trial of the American Association for the Surgery of Trauma. *J of Trauma.* 1997; 42 (3): 375-380.
4. Parmley LF, Amnion WC, Mattingly TW. Non-penetrating traumatic injury of the heart. *Circulation.* 1958; 17: 1086-1101.
5. Smith MD, Cassidy JM, Souther S, et al. Transesophageal echocardiography in the diagnosis of traumatic rupture of the aorta. *N Eng J Med.* 1995; 332-356.
6. Gavant ML, Menke PG, Fabian TC, et al. Blunt traumatic aortic rupture: Detection with helical CT of the chest. *Radiology.* 1995; 197:125.
7. Miller FB, Richardson JD, Thomas HA, et al. Role of CT in the diagnosis of major arterial injury after blunt thoracic trauma. *Surgery.* 1989; 106-596.
8. Mattox KL, Holzman M. Pickard LR, et al. Clamp/repair: A safe technique for treatment of blunt injury to the descending thoracic aorta. *Ann Thorac Surg.* 1985; 40 (5): 456-462.
9. Akins CW, Buckley MJ, Daggett W, et al. Acute traumatic disruption of the thoracic aorta: A ten year experience. *Ann Thorac Surg.* 1980; 31: 305.
10. Verdant AG, Mercier CH, Page AA, et al. Aneurysm of the descending thoracic aorta: Treatment with the Gott shunt. *Can J Surg.* 1981; 24: 594.
11. Wellons ED, Milner R, Solis M, et al. Stent-graft repair of thoracic aortic disruptions. *J Vasc Surg.* 2004; 40: 1095-1100.
12. Symbus PN. Sherman AJ, Silver JM, et al. Traumatic rupture of the aorta: Immediate or delayed repair? *Ann Surg.* 2002; 235 (6): 796-802.
13. Daenen G, Maleux G, Daenent K, et al. Thoracic aorta endoprosthesis: The final countdown for open surgery after traumatic aortic rupture? *Ann Vasc Surg.* 2003; 17: 185-191.
14. Rosenthal D, Wellons E, Birkett A, et al. Endovascular repair of traumatic thoracic aortic disruption with "stacked" abdominal endograft extension cuffs. *J Vasc Surg.* 2008; 48 (4): 841-844.
15. Rousseau H, Danebrin C, Marcheix B, et al. Acute traumatic aortic rupture: A comparison of surgical and stent-graft repair. *J of Thorac and Cardiovasc Surg.* 2005; 129 (5): 1050-1055.
16. Neschis D, Moaine S, Gutta R, et al. Twenty consecutive cases of endograft repair of traumatic aortic disruption: Lessons learned. *J Vasc Surg.* 2007; 45: 487-492.
17. Hoornweg LL, Dinkelman MK, Goslings JC, et al. Endovascular management of traumatic ruptures of the thoracic aorta: A retrospective multicenter analysis of 28 cases in the Netherlands. *J Vasc Surg.* 2006; 43 (6): 1096.
18. Hirose H, Gill I, Malangoni M. Nonoperative management of traumatic aortic injury. *The J of Trauma Injury, Infection and Critical Care.* 2006; 60: 5979-601.
19. Fisher R, Oria R, Ki M, et al. Conservative management of aortic lacerations due to blunt trauma. *J of Trauma.* 1990; 30: 1562-1566.
20. Kepros J, Angood P, Jaffe C, Rabinovici R. Aortic intimal injuries from blunt trauma: Resolution profile in nonoperative management. *J of Trauma.* 2002; 52: 475-478.
21. Langanay T, Verhoye JP, Corbineau H, et al. Surgical treatment of acute traumatic rupture of the thoracic aorta of timing reappraisal. *Eur J Cardiothorac Surg.* 2002; 21 (2): 282-287.

22. Maggigano R, Nathans A, Alexandrova NA, et al. Traumatic rupture of the thoracic aorta: Should one always operate immediately? *Ann Vasc Surg.* 1995; 9: 44-52.

23. Pacini D, Angeli E, Fattori R, et al. Traumatic rupture of the thoracic aorta: Ten years of delayed management. *J Thorac Cardiovasc Surg.* 2005; 129: 880-884.

24. Pate JW, Fabian TC, Walker WA. Traumatic rupture of the aortic isthmus: An emergency? *World J Surg.* 1995; 19: 119-120.

25. Kipfer B, Leupi F, Scheupback P, et al. Traumatic rupture of the thoracic aorta: Immediate or delayed surgical repair? *Eur J Cardiothorac Surgery.* 1994; 8:30-33.

26. Reed AB, Thompson JK. Timing of endovascular repair of traumatic aortic transections. *J Vasc Surg.* 2006; 43 (4): 684.

27. Kieffer E, Leschi J. Chiche L. Open repair of chronic post-traumatic aneurysm of the aortic isthmus: The value of direct aortoaortic anastomosis. *J Vasc Surg.* 2005; 41: 931-935.

28. Stampfl P, Greitbauer M. Zimpfer D, et al. Mid-term results of conservative, conventional and endovascular treatment for acute traumatic aortic lesions. *Eur J of Vasc and Endovasc surg.* 2006; 31 (5): 475.

29. Finkelmeier B, Mentzer RJ, Kaiser D, et al. Chronic traumatic thoracic aneurysm. Influence of operative treatment on nature history: An analysis of reported cases, 1950-1980. *J Thorac Cardiovasc Surg.* 1982; 84: 257-266.

30. Kasirajan K, Heffernan D, Langsfeld M. Acute thoracic aorta trauma: A comparison of endoluminal stent grafts with open repair and nonoperative management. *Ann of Vasc Surg.* 2003; 17: 489-595.

31. Ott M, Stewart T, Lawlor D, et al. Management of blunt thoracic aortic injuries: Endovascular stents versus open repair. *J of Trauma.* 2004; 56: 565-570.

32. McCollum C, Graham J, Noon G, DeBakey M. Chronic traumatic aneurysm of the thoracic aorta: An analysis of 50 patients. *J of Trauma.* 1979; 19: 248- 252.

33. Lebl D, Dicker R, Spain D, Brundage S. Dramatic shift in the primary management of traumatic thoracic aortic rupture. *Arch Surgery.* 2006; 141: 177-180.

34. Kieffer E. Chiche L, Lormier E, Guegan H. Recurrent spinal cord ischemia after endovascular stent graft for chronic traumatic aneurysm of the aortic isthmus. *J of Vasc Surg.* 2007; 45 (4): 831.

35. Stevens SL, Farber MA, eds. *Thoracic endovascular aorta.* Knoxville, TN: Tennessee Valley Publishing; 2008.

36. Ryan M, Valazquez O, Martine E, et al. Thoracic aortic transection treated by thoracic endovascular aortic repair: Predictors of survival. *Vasc and Endovasc Surg.* 2010; 44 (2): 95-100.

37. Diethrich EB, Ramaiah VG, Kpodona J. Rodriguez-Lopez JA. *Endovascular and hybrid management of the thoracic aorta.* Hoboken, NJ: Blackwell Publishing; 2008.

38. Lumsden AB, Lin PH, Chen C, Parody JC. *Advanced endovascular therapy of aortic disease.* Malden, MA: Blackwell Publishing; 2007.

39. Katz M, Blackstone E, Kirklin J, et al. incremental risk factors for spinal cord injury following operation for acute traumatic aortic transection. *J. Thorac Cardiovasc Surg.* 1981; 81: 669.

40. Borsa JJ, Hhoffer, EK, Karmy-Jones R, et al. Angiographic description of blunt traumatic injuries to the thoracic aorta with specific relevance to endographic repair. *J Enderas Ther.* 2002; 9 (suppl 2): 1184-1191.

41. Ehrlich MP, Rousseau H, Heijam R, et al. early outcome of endovascular treatment of acute traumatic aortic injuries: The talent thoracic retrospective registry. *Ann Thorac Surg.* 2009; 88: 1258.

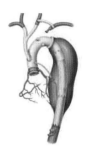

CHAPTER 11

Repair of an Extensive Thoracic Aortic Aneurysm with Debranching, Antegrade Endograft Delivery, and use of a Customized Collar-Graft

Extensive thoracic aortic aneurysms involving the ascending, transverse, and descending thoracic aorta have traditionally been repaired using the elephant-trunk technique as described by Hans Borst in 1983.[1] The operative mortality is reported at 2% to 12% for Stage-One and 3.9% to 9.6% for Stage-Two. In addition, there is a significant attrition rate with a 16% mortality risk between the stages.[2-5] The use of hybrid endografting procedures has, in some cases, allowed such extensive thoracic aneurysms to be repaired in one stage.

The Polyester Siena Graft was developed by Vascutek Corporation. The Siena graft has a collar affixed to the body of the graft and is available from the manufacturer in a number of configurations. The collar can be trimmed to size to compensate for diameter discrepancies along the length of the aorta. The anastomosis of the collar to the aorta replaces the invaginated graft anastomosis of the traditional elephant-trunk. Recently, the vastitude Company has produced a customized collar graft to my specifications and shown in figure 11-1. The

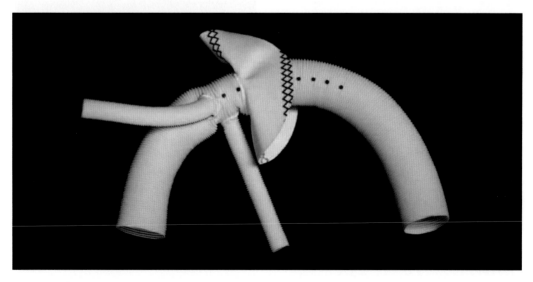

Figure 11-1 Customized Siena graft with radiopaque markers, collar, and lateral sideport for antegrade endograft delivery.

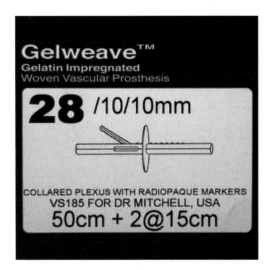

Figure 11-2 Customized collared plexus graft.

lower medial sidearm can be used for arterial inflow from the cardiopulmonary bypass circuit. The lateral 10 mm sidearm is at a 90° angle from the first sidearm and at a 30° takeoff angle from the body of the graft. This lateral sidearm will accommodate a 24-Fr sheath and facilitates antegrade delivery of a thoracic endograft, figure 11-2. The placement and angle of this sidearm allows the endograft to follow the natural curve of the aortic arch. Additionally, the endograft can be deployed via the lateral sidearm while maintaining cardiopulmonary bypass and re-warming via the medial sidearm. Obviously, femoral arterial in-flow would be unsatisfactory with the distal trunk of the graft free in the descending aorta. The graft is manufactured with radiopaque markers at 2 cm intervals for fluoroscopic visualization and measuring overlap should endografts be deployed within the Siena graft.

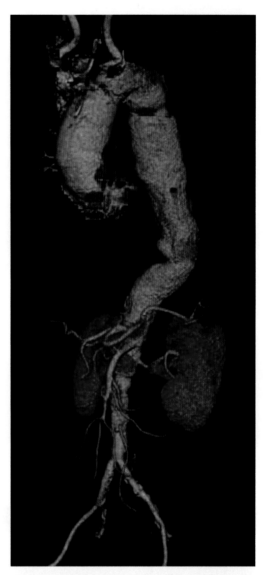

Figure 11-3 CT angiogram of thoracic aortic aneurysm, preoperative. Note small iliac arteries.

There is another advantage of the collar-graft that makes it uniquely suited to hybrid endograft procedures. As Dacron is known to expand over time, endografts placed within Dacron should be oversized by at least 20%.[6] By using a collar-graft, a smaller graft body can be chosen to optimize seal with the endograft while the collar itself compensates for the size of the aorta at the hand-sutured anastomosis. Once the distal end of the endograft (proximal end with antegrade delivery) is landed in the native aorta, the collar-to-aorta anastomosis becomes inconsequential as it is pressurized only by back-bleeding intercostal arteries from the excluded aneurysm sac.

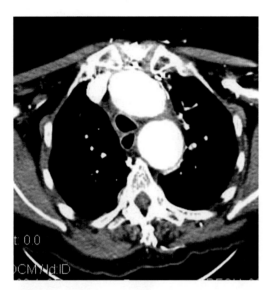

Figure 11-4 Axial CT image of thoracic aortic aneurysm, preoperative.

CASE SCENARIO:
Debranching of Thoracic Aneurysms and Antegrade ELG Delivery

A 65-year-old patient presented with an acute my-ocardial infarction and underwent angioplasty and stenting to a culprit lesion in the right coronary ar-tery. The patient was diagnosed with a 70% steno-sis in the circumflex coronary artery, aortic valvular stenosis, and an extensive thoracic aortic aneurysm involving the ascending, transverse, and descend-ing thoracic aorta as seen in figures 11-3 and 11-4.

The repair of this thoracic aortic aneurysm began by debranching the left subclavian artery with a left carotid to left subclavian bypass using an 8 mm polytetrafluoroethylene graft. Such large thoracic aortic aneurysms will tend to displace the origin of the left subclavian artery far into the left chest, which adds difficulty in dealing with the left subclavian artery via a median sternotomy approach. The right axillary artery was exposed to use for both cardiopulmonary bypass and ante-grade cerebral perfusion. After median sternotomy, the patient was cooled to electroencephalographic silence via right axillary artery and right atrial

cardiopulmonary bypass. During cooling, a saphe-nous vein graft was used to bypass the stenotic circumflex coronary artery and the aortic valve was replaced with a prosthetic tissue valve. The aortic sinus and root were acceptable and the coronary ostia were not re-implanted as a conduit.

The base of the innominate artery was clamped and the aortic arch was opened while maintaining cerebral perfusion via the right axillary artery. Back-bleeding was noted from the origin of the left carotid artery, confirming the intact circle of Willis which we knew from preoperative arteriography.

One limb of a bifurcated graft was sutured to the left carotid artery. A second clamp was applied to one limb of the bifurcated graft and a 20-Fr arterial cannula was placed in the main body of the bifurcated graft. This allowed arterial in-flow directly via both the left carotid and right axillary artery while the anastomosis to the base of the innominate was constructed to the other limb of the bifurcated graft.

The circulatory arrest time with no antegrade flow directly into the left carotid artery was only seven minutes, but during that seven minutes there was antegrade flow via the right axillary artery to the cerebral vasculature. Thus, there was 0 minutes of no cerebral flow during head vessel revascular-ization. A size 30 mm customized Siena graft was placed in the descending thoracic aorta as an elephant-trunk and the collar sutured to the aorta. The proximal end of the Siena graft was sutured to the native aortic tissue just above the newly implanted valve. The medial sidearm of the customized collar-graft was cannulated for re-warming the body as the bifurcated graft was sutured low on the lateral wall of the collar-graft, as illustrated in figure 11-5.

Two 37 mm thoracic endografts were delivered antegrade via the lateral 10 mm sidearm of the customized collar-graft. The endografts landed a few centimeters above the celiac artery, as illustrated in figure 11-6. Radiopaque markers on the collar-graft facilitate intraoperative measurements of overlap of the

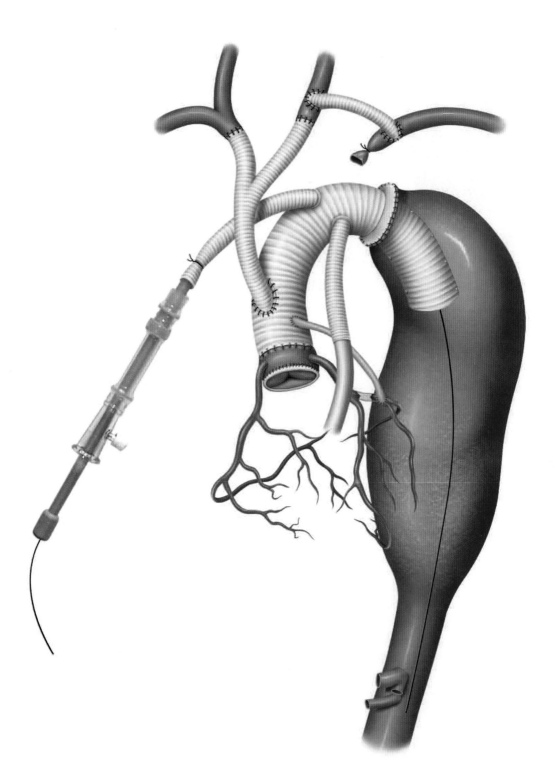

Figure 11-5 Use of the customized collar Siena graft with lateral sidearm for endograft delivery.

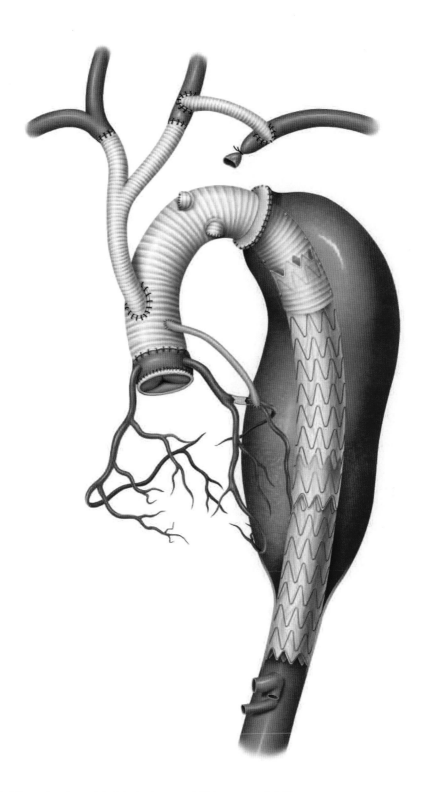

Figure 11-6 Illustration of completed single-stage repair. Sidearms now tied off.

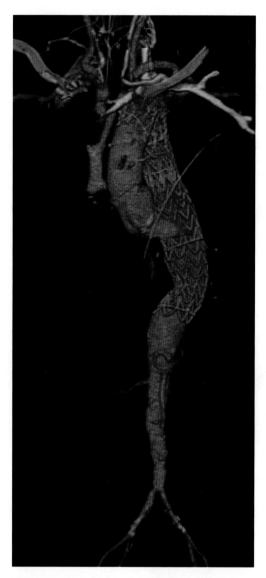

Figure 11-7 CT angiogram of completed repair. Note the small iliac arteries would have prevented retrograde ELG delivery.

endograft into the collar-graft. This allows single stage correction of extensive thoracic aortic aneurysms while maintaining antegrade cerebral flow. Figure 11-7 demonstrates the postoperative repair. Note the small iliac arteries would have prevented retrograde endograft delivery.

COMMENTARY

(Edward B. Diethrich, Phoenix, AZ) This case illustrates the ultimate capacity for the hybrid procedural concept to treat complex combined aortic valvular and aneurysmal pathology. The use of the customized collar Siena grafts, described with instructions from Dr. Mitchell, adds the unique feature to the technique. The procedure also depicts the concept of antegrade endoluminal graft delivery which we described earlier in a case of type I dissection. The major advantage of the antegrade delivery is to overcome problems of retrograde femoral artery delivery in the presence of either small or diseased vessels. A 240 cm wire can be passed through the 10 mm delivery sheath on the ascending aorta and exteriorized at the common femoral artery. This allows tension to be placed on the wire like a banjo string, enhancing the smooth passage of the endoluminal grafts across the aortic arch to the descending thoracic aorta. The concept is illustrated well in another case in chapter 15.

REFERENCES

1. Borst HG, Waltersbusch G, Schaps D. Extensive aortic replacement using "elephant trunk" prosthesis. *Thoracic Cardiovascular Surgery.* 1983; 31 (1): 37-40.

2. Estrera AL, Miller III CC, Chen EP, et al. Descending Thoracic Aortic Aneurysm Repair: 12-year experience using distal aortic perfusion and cerebrospinal fluid drainage. *Ann Thoracic Surg.* 2005; 80 (4): 1290.

3. Safi HJ, Miller III CC, Etrera AL et al. Optimization of aortic arch replacement: two-stage approach. *Ann Thoracic Surg.* 2007; 83 (2): S 815-818.

4. Svensson LG, Kim KH, Blackstone E H, et al. Elephant-truck procedure: newer indication and uses. *Ann Thoracic Surg.* 2004; 78 (1): 109-116.

5. Lemaire SA, Carter SA, Coselli, JS. The elephant-trunk technique for staged repair of the entire thoracic aorta. *Ann Thoracic Surg.* 2006; 81 (5): 1561-1569.

6. Hughes GC, Nienaber JJ, Bush EL, et al. Use of custom Dacron branch grafts for "hybrid" aortic debranching during endovascular repair of thoracic and thoracoabdominal aortic aneurysms. *J of Thoracic and Cardiovascular Surg.* 2008; 136: 21-28.

CHAPTER 12

Endovascular Repair of a Transverse Aortic Arch Aneurysm with Debranching and Retrograde Carotid Artery Chimney Grafts

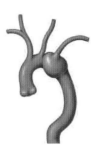

Currently, thoracic endovascular aortic repair (TEVAR) devices are only approved by the United States Food and Drug Administration for deployment in landing zones 2 and 3. Landing zones 2 and 3 are proximal and distal to the origin of the left subclavian artery, respectively, as seen in figure 12-1.[1] The placement of an endograft in zone 2 will, by definition, occlude the left subclavian artery. This may or may not require the use of a carotid artery to left subclavian artery bypass. Because the origin of the left carotid and left subclavian arteries are often in very close proximity, aneurysms or dissections involving the origin of the left subclavian artery may require coverage of the left carotid artery to obtain adequate seal and to prevent endoleaks. The region of the aortic arch immediately proximal to the left carotid origin is landing zone 1, figure 12-1.[1]

In situations of either intentional or inadvertent encroachment of the left carotid artery, the surgeon must be familiar with strategies to manage this very unforgiving problem. As custom-made branched grafts are not yet commercially available, a number of other techniques have evolved. Treatment options including debranching procedures with or without extra-anatomic bypass, chimney or snorkel grafts, and in situ fenestration.[2-9]

Debranching procedures involve placing

grafts from the ascending aorta to one or more head vessels with subsequent endografting the aortic arch to cover the origin of the de/rebranched arteries. This technique has been described both with and without the use of extra-anatomic bypass procedures. Chapters 13 and 15 detail hybrid de/rebranching techniques used in the aortic arch.

In situ fenestration is an interesting technique reported Sonesson and Malina.[9] A temporary femoral to bicarotid artery bypass is constructed to

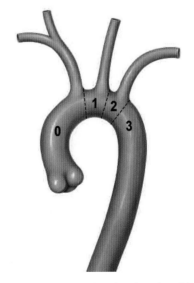

Figure 12-1 Numerical location of aortic endograft landing zones.[1]

provide blood flow to the brain. The transverse aortic arch can then be endografted to exclude the origin of the innominate and left carotid/subclavian arteries. Working retrograde through each carotid artery, but below the temporary bypass conduit, the thoracic graft is punctured with a spinal needle to gain wire access. A hole or fenestration in the thoracic graft is serially dilated until a stent can be passed retrograde from the innominate artery and left carotid artery into the thoracic endograft. This essentially results in a branched-thoracic endograft with the branches supplying blood to the head vessels. The temporary femoral to bicarotid artery bypass is then removed or inactivated.

Although these hybrid and endovascular techniques offer an early reduction in perioperative mortality and morbidity when compared with traditional open-surgery, the long-term durability of these procedures is unknown. However, for the elderly and those patients with significant comorbidities, these minimally invasive alternatives may be life-saving.

The below case scenario describes a patient with a thoracic aortic aneurysm involving the origin of the left subclavian artery. TEVAR was complicated by occlusion of the left carotid artery.

CASE SCENARIO:
Carotid artery chimney grafts

A 75-year-old man presented with a thoracic aortic aneurysm involving the base of the left subclavian artery. The proximal extent of the aneurysm extended to very near the distal aspect of the left common carotid artery origin, as illustrated in figure 12-2. There was a calcified dissection plane identified within the aneurysm by computerized tomography. This indicates a probable localized chronic dissection that had become aneurysmal over time.

Under general anesthesia, the right femoral artery was identified by cutdown and a 24-Fr sheath was advanced into the abdominal aorta over a stiff 0.035 inch guide wire. A TAG endoprosthesis size 34 mm x 10 cm was deployed within the thoracic aorta and insufflated with a tri-lobed balloon. Intraoperative arteriogram, figure 12-3, demonstrates exclusion of the aneurysm with no endoleak. The left subclavian artery was occluded by the endograft as expected. Initially, it appeared that the left carotid artery was opacified by contrast agent. However, on close inspection, there was a paucity of contrast in the left carotid artery as compared to the innominate artery. In addition, it

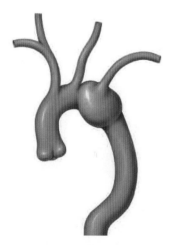

Figure 12-2 Illustration of thoracic aortic aneurysm with proximity to landing zone 1.

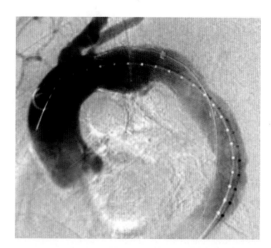

Figure 12-3 Intraoperative arteriogram. Note graft encroachment on left carotid artery and paucity of contrast agent in left carotid compared with innominate artery. The left subclavian artery is excluded.

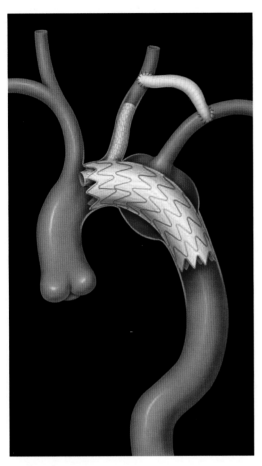

Figure 12-4 Illustration of chimney graft, thoracic endograft and carotid to left subclavian artery bypass.

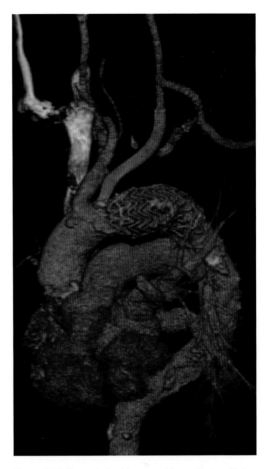

Figure 12-5 Computerized tomographic angiogram. Note relationship of chimney graft to thoracic endograft. The carotid to subclavian artery bypass remains patent.

appeared a proximal flange from the endograft was partially occluding the left carotid artery. A subsequent cutdown on the left carotid artery revealed no palpable pulse and a pressure-monitor catheter demonstrated an 80 mm pressure gradient between the left carotid artery and the right radial artery.

Under Fluoroscopic guidance, a 0.035 inch guide wire was placed retrograde from the left carotid artery into the ascending aorta. Through a 9-Fr introducer sheath, a 9 mm diameter x 10 cm covered Viabahn graft was deployed in retrograde fashion into the aorta via the left carotid artery. The aortic end of the chimney/snorkel graft was positioned 0.5 cm past the proximal end of the thoracic aortic endograft. The distal end of the chimney graft remained in the left common carotid artery. In addition, a left carotid to left subclavian bypass was then constructed using a 6 mm ringed, heparin-bonded polytetrafluoroethylene Propaten graft. The completed procedure is illustrated in figure 12-4. At 18 months follow-up, the aneurysm remains repaired and the patient has no neurologic deficits or arm claudication. Computerized tomographic angiography demonstrates aneurysm exclusion and the relationships of the carotid artery chimney graft to the main body thoracic endograft. The carotid to subclavian artery bypass remains patent at 18 months post operatively, figure 12-5.

REFERENCES

1. Ishimaru S. Endografting of the Aortic Arch. *Journal Endovascular Ther.* 2004; 11: II-62-II-71.

2. Riesenman PJ, Tamaddon HS, Farber MA. *Surgical Bypass Procedures to Facilitate Endovascular Repair of Aortic Arch Pathology.*

3. Hughes GC, Nienaber JJ, Bush EL, et al. Use of Custom Dacron Branch Grafts for "Hybrid" Aortic Debranching during Endovascular Repair of Thoracic and Thoracoabdominal Aortic Aneurysms. *Journal of Thoracic Cardiovascular Surgery.* 2008; 136: 21-28.

4. Mitchell RO, Rogers AG, Earle G, Imam M. Hybrid Endovascular Repair of Thoracic Aortic Aneurysms by Debranching and the Creation of Landing Zone-Zero. *Journal Kentucky Medical Association.* 2009; Vol 107 (11): 438-441.

5. Criado FJ. Pushing the Envelope with Complex TEVAR. *Endovascular Today.* 2007; Nov: 11-18.

6. Baldwin ZK, Chuter T AM, Hiramoto JS, et al. Double-barrel Technique for Preservation of Aortic Arch Branches during Thoracic Endovascular Aortic Repair. *Ann Vascular Surgery.* 2008; 22: 703-709.

7. Criado FJ. A Percutaneous Technique for Preservation of Arch Branch Patency During Thoracic Endovascular Aortic Repair (TEVAR). *Journal Endovascular Ther.* 2007; 14:54-58.

8. Wang GJ and Woo EY. Snorkel Procedure for TEVAR. *Journal Endovascular Ther.* 2009; 8 (10): 48-51.

9. Sonesson B, Resch T, Allers M. Malina M. Endovascular Total Aortic Arch Replacement by In Situ Stent Graft Fenestration Technique. *Journal Vascular Surgery.* 2009; 49: 1589-91.

CHAPTER 13

Hybrid Endovascular Repair of Extensive Thoracic Aortic Aneurysms by Debranching and the Creation of Landing Zone-Zero

Advances in minimally invasive thoracic endo-grafting techniques have significantly reduced the perioperative mortality of descending thoracic aneurysm repair. In one study, 105 patients with thoracic aneurysms were treated with either open-surgery or endovascular repair. The 30-day mortality was 7.6% versus 15.1% for the endovascular and open repair groups, respectively (P = 0.09).[1]

In a study from the Netherlands, 42 patients with thoracic aneurysms were treated with endo- or open-surgery. The mortality rate was 5% and 11% in the endo and open groups, respectively (P = 0.33).[2]

The multicenter GORE TAG pivotal trial compared 140 patients treated with endografts and 94 patients treated with open surgery. The 30-day mortality was 2.1% in the endovascular group versus 11.7% in the open group (P = 0.001).[3] The Medtronic Talent graft demonstrated similarly superior results when compared with open surgery in the VALOR trial.[4] These trials consisted of patients with isolated descending TAAs.

However, an even greater surgical challenge than isolated descending thoracic aneurysms are those aneurysms that involve the transverse aortic arch. Transverse arch aneurysms demand particular attention be paid to the supra-aortic arch vessels. Traditional open repair has required hypothermic circulatory assent and/or cerebral perfusion while the innominate and carotid arter-

ies are reimplanted by hand suturing into a graft. In some series the mortality for open transverse arch aneurysm repair approaches 25%.[5]

Two considerations for the endovascular repair of transverse arch aneurysms involve first acquiring an area of normal aorta proximal to the aneurysm to serve as a "landing-zone" for the endograft to maintain firm attachment. Secondly, any great vessel arising from the aortic arch that will be occluded by the endograft must be revascularized prior to endograft deployment. A variety of debranching and revascularization strategies have been proposed. These included carotid-to-carotid bypass, carotid-to-subclavian transposition, and femoral-to-axillary-to-carotid bypass.[6,7]

Available landing zones for endografts have been described.[8] The least commonly used landing zone is zone-zero. Zone-zero lies proximal to the innominate artery and an endograft deployed in the zone would occlude the origin of all the arch vessels: the innominate, right and left carotid, and right and left subclavian arteries. Extensive re-branching techniques are required to revascularize all of these arch vessels. The usual rebranching method involves suturing a bifurcated graft low on the ascending aorta (zone-zero) and using this graft to revascularize the innominate and carotid arteries. Fewer than 50 of these procedures have been reported in the English language literature.[4,7,9-11]

Even more unusual than using the native landing zone-zero is the actual creation of the landing zone-zero when none existed. I have called this neo-zone-zero. In the patient described below, I outline the hybrid management of a complex aneurysm involving the ascending, transverse, and descending aorta by the creation of neo-zone-zero to serve as both a source of rebranching and proximal endograft fixation.

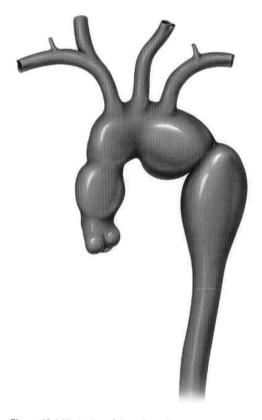

Figure 13-1 Illustration of thoracic aortic aneurysm involving the ascending, transverse, and proximal descending aorta.

CASE SCENARIO:
Creating Zone-Zero

The patient is a 72-year-old man with a complex thoracic aortic aneurysm involving the ascending, transverse, and descending thoracic aorta, figure 13-1. The patient had previously undergone surgi-

cal resection of an esophageal cancer. His aneurysm had been followed closely until the transverse component approached 6 cm and he was 6 years post esophageal resection with no evidence of tumor recurrence by positron emission tomography.

Under general anesthesia and with continuous electro-encephalographic (EEG) monitoring, a median sternotomy was performed. The patient was placed on normothermic cardiopulmonary bypass via the right femoral artery and right atrial appendage. The ascending aortic aneurysm was replaced with a 32 mm Dacron graft to create landing zone-zero. The Dacron graft had pre-attached 8 and 10 mm sidearms. The innominate artery was selectively clamped. As no EEG changes were noted, the innominate artery was transected from the native aortic arch and sutured in end-to-end fashion to the 10 mm Dacron side-arm. Similarly, the left carotid artery was transected and sutured to the 8 mm side-arm.

The use of continuous EEG monitoring allowed the avoidance of hypothermic circulatory arrest. As the right vertebral artery was large and the circle of Willis intact, as demonstrated by pre-op arteriography, the left subclavian artery could be ligated with minimal risk of a verte-brobasilar stroke. The lateral displacement of the left subclavian artery made its management difficult from a median sternotomy incision. A pre-procedure left carotid to subclavian bypass should be considered when the origin of the left subclavian artery is displaced laterally.

Finally, a section of radiopaque marking wire was attached to the ascending Dacron graft just about the origin of the sidearms. This would serve as a fluoroscopic warning marking during placement of the endograft. If the endograft were deployed below this marking ring, the sidearms supplying the great vessels would be occluded.

Using the left femoral artery as an access site, two TAG thoracic endografts, size 34 mm by 20 cm, were deployed within neo-zone-zero to completely exclude the aneurysm, figure 13-2. Note occasionally the endografts may be deployed from within the chest in an antegrade fashion, see Chapter 15.

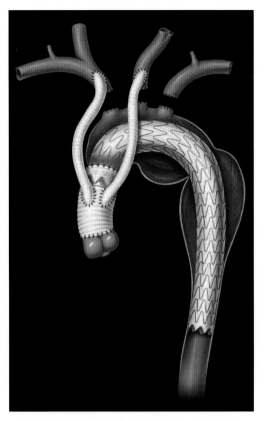

Figure 13-2 Illustration of repaired thoracic aneurysm with Dacron ascending graft to create neo-zone-zero, debranched cerebral vessels, and endograft excluding aneurysm.

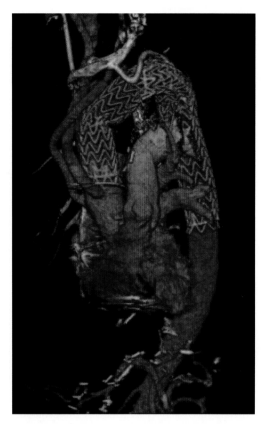

Figure 13-3 Computerize tomography 18 months post procedure. Note the proximal Dacron graft and the two sidearms do not appear "white" in this scan as they contain no metal.

However, in this case, the deployment site was so proximal in the ascending graft, that the retrograde femoral approach seemed more reasonable. In addition, it is somewhat more difficult to place the hub of the endograft with the precision that can be achieved at the tip end. In this case, extreme accuracy was needed to have maximum endograft overlays within neo-zone-zero and still not occlude the sidearms.

Figure 13-3 demonstrates continued graft patency, absence of endoleak or graft migration, and patency of the rebranching conduit sidearms at 18 months post procedure. Just prior to three year follow-up the patient expired from metastatic melanoma.

CASE DISCUSSION:
Creating Zone-Zero

Thoracic endografting and hybrid techniques are continuing to evolve and offer a mortality advantage over open surgical repairs. Although extended-term durability statistics are lacking, this case demonstrates the durability of a hybrid repair of a complex thoracic aneurysm by the creation of a neo-zone-zero to function as an endograft landing site. Electroencephalographic guidance and sequential debranching technique allowed for the successful repair of this complicated aneurysm without the need of circulatory arrest or selective cerebral perfusion strategies. Endografts placed within Dacron grafts should be oversized to compensate for Dacron expansion over time.[12]

REFERENCES

1. Stone OH, Brewster DC, Kuolek CJ, et al. Stent Graft Versus Open Surgical Repair of the Thoracic Aorta: Midterm Results. *Journal of Vascular Surgery*. 2006; 44 (6): 1188.

2. Glade GH, Vahl AC, Wisselink W. Mid-term Survival and Cost of Treatment of Patients With Descending Thoracic Aneurysms; Endovascular vs. Open Repair; A Case-Controlled Study. *European Journal of Vascular and Endovascular Surgery*. 2005; 29 (1): 28-34.

3. Bavaria JE, Appoo JJ, Makaroun MS, et al. Endovascular Stent Grafting Versus Open Surgical Repair of Descending Thoracic Aneurysms In Low-Risk Patients: A Multicenter Comparative Trial. *Journal of Thoracic and Cardiovascular Surgery*. 2007; 133 (2): 369.

4. Fairman RM, Criado F, Farber M, et al. Pivotal Results of the Medtronic Vascular Talent Thoracic Stent Graft System: The VALVOR Trial. *Journal of Vascular Surgery*. 2008; 48: 546-54.

5. Bergeron P, Mungialardi N, Costa P, et al. Great Vessel Management for Endovascular Exclusion of Aortic Arch Aneurysms and Dissections. *European Journal of Vascular and Endovascular Surgery*. 2006; 32: 38-45.

6. Criado F, Clark NS Barnatan MF Stent Graft Repair in the Aortic Arch and Descending Aorta: A Four Year Experience. *Journal of Vascular Surgery*. 2002; 36 (6): 1121-1128.

7. Shemming W, Guangic C, Xiaoxi L, et al. Endovascular Treatment of Arch and Proximal Thoracic Aortic Lesions. *Journal of Vascular Surgery*. 2009: 48 (1) 64-68.

8. Ishimaru S. Endografting the Aortic Arch. *Journal of Endovascular Therapy*. 2004; 11: II-62-II-71.

9. Saleh HM, Inglese L. Combined Surgical and Endovascular Treatment of Aortic Arch Aneurysms. *Journal of Vascular Surgery*. 1998 Nov; 5 (4): 329-332.

10. Zhou W, Reardon M, Peden EK, et al. Hybrid Approach to Complex Thoracic Aortic Aneurysms In High Risk Patients. Surgical Challenges and Clinical Outcomes. *Journal of Vascular Surgery*. 2006 Oct; 44 (4): 688-693.

11. Stevens SL, Farber MA, eds. *Thoracic Endovascular Aorta*. Knoxville, TN: Tennessee Valley Publishing; 2008.

12. Hughes GC, Nienaber JJ, Bush EL, et al. Use of Custom Dacron Branch Grafts for "Hybrid" Aortic Descending During Endovascular Repair of Thoracic and Thoracoabdominal Aortic Aneurysm. *Journal of Thoracic and Cardiovascular Surgery*. 2008; 136; 21-28.

CHAPTER 14

Endograft Repair of Type B Aortic Dissection with Five and a Half Year Follow-Up

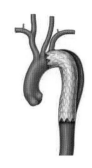

Longitudinal tears in the aortic wall that originate distal to the left subclavian artery are classified as Stanford type-B aortic dissections. The incidence of aortic dissections in the United States is approximately 10,000 cases annually.[1] The in-hospital mortality for type B dissections managed medically is 10%; whereas open surgery for complicated dissections has a mortality of 31%.[2,3] These mortality statistics have resulted in most patients receiving medical therapy, which consists primarily of aggressive blood pressure control and finger-crossing. Intravenous beta-blockers reduce the pulsatile force (dp/dt) within the aorta and theoretically reduces the progression of dissection. Open surgery has been reserved for those patients developing complications of the dissection such as rupture, visceral or limb ischemia, or enlargement. These very complications that provide an indication for open surgery also portend a poor operative outcome.

Although medical therapy may initially seem to provide a favorable outcome in uncomplicated dissections, the intermediate and long-term results are not nearly as satisfying. Within three years of hospital discharge, one in four patients will be dead.[4] Within 10 years of hospital discharge, survival with a type B dissection is just over 40%.[4,6]

The endograft treatment of complicated dissections has been reported to have a 5.3% mortality at 30 days.[7] This is favorable when compared to the open surgical mortality of 30% for complicated dissections. However, in the case of uncomplicated dissections, endografting does not demonstrate an early survival advantage compared to medical therapy.

The INSTEAD trial randomized patients with uncomplicated, stable type B dissections into receiving either endovascular surgery or best medical therapy. At one year, there was no statistical survival advantage in either group.[8] Although it might be expected that the endograft group would demonstrate a survival benefit at a longer term, that data is not yet available.

At this time is can be concluded that endografting offers a substantial survival benefit when compared to open surgery in the case of complicated dissections. The role of endografting in stable, uncomplicated dissections remains unclear. As of yet, there is no endograft currently approved by the Food and Drug Administration for treating type B dissections in the United States.

CASE SCENARIO:
Type B Dissection

The patient is a 71-year-old woman who present with 48 hours of severe interscapular pain. Computerize tomographic (CT) scanning demonstrated a type B aortic dissection extending from

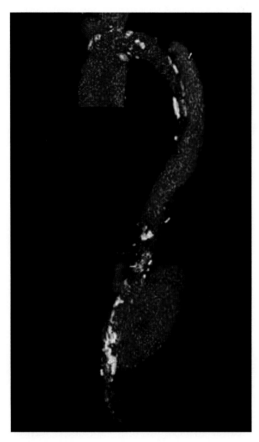

Figure 14-1 Computerized Tomography of type B aortic dissection.

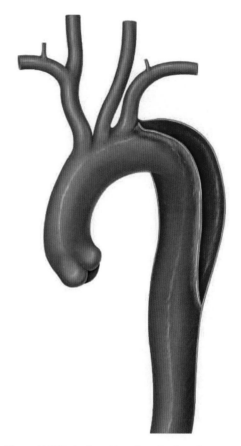

Figure 14-2 Illustration of type B aortic dissection.

the left subclavian artery to the aortic hiatus at the diaphragm, figure 14-1. Figure 14-2 illustrates these findings. The patient was initially managed medially but returned in approximately 3 weeks with continued pain and aneurysmal enlargement. Endograft therapy was offered as a treatment option. The patient and family were fully informed that this was an "off-label" therapy and that "open" surgery was an alternative.

Under general anesthesia, the right femoral artery was identified by cutdown. Using a 24-Fr delivery sheath, a 37 mm by 20 cm TAG endograft was deployed in the thoracic aorta. Intraaortic ultrasound is an invaluable tool to ensure graft deployment in the true-lumen of the dissection. In difficult cases, a wire from the right brachial artery

into the ascending aorta or left ventricle can be snared to ensure true lumen access proximally. Unlike endografts used to treat true aneurysms, balloon insufflations should be avoided in the case of dissections as the dissection may propagate retrograde into the transverse or ascending aorta.

Figure 14-3 demonstrates the initial postoperative repair. Note that the endograft proximally directs antegrade aortic blood flow into the true lumen, but a distal area of dissections remains. I chose not to cover this area as such long-segment coverage would increase the risk of paralysis, and the properly directed blood flow would likely obliterate the false lumen over time. Figure 14-4 illustrates the repair. Figures 14-5 a, b, c, d are CT images at 12, 24, 36, and 66 months post repair,

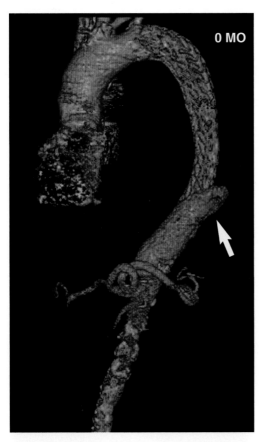

Figure 14-3 Computerized tomography immediately following endograft repair of a type B aortic dissection. Note: Residual distal false lumen, white arrow.

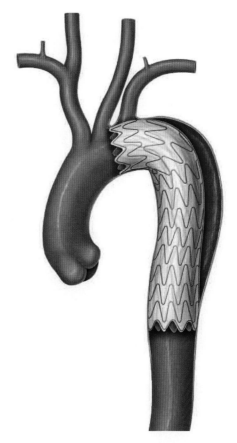

Figure 14-4 Illustration of endograft repair of type B dissection.

respectively. The scan at 12 months demonstrates resolution of the distal false lumen. The scan at 66 months demonstrates the durability of the repair with no evidence of stent migration, aneurysmal enlargement, endoleak, or residual false lumen.

CASE DISCUSSION:
Type B Dissection

Type B aortic dissections have remained a difficult management problem. Open surgical techniques have had a very high periopetative mortality, and medical therapy has not produced satisfactory long-term results. Endovascular grafting techniques may provide a favorable alternative to open surgical therapy. At this time there are no endo-grafts approved by the U.S. Food and Drug Administration for treating type B dissections. Also, there is very little data on the long-term efficiency of endovascular stents used "off-label" to treat dissections. The surgeon managing such maladies must be versed in distinguishing acute versus chronic and complicated versus uncompli-cated dissections, as well as the use of intravascular ultrasound.

The above case scenario illustrates that complicated aortic dissections can be successfully treated by minimally invasive endograft techniques in a community hospital. In addition, the serial follow-up demonstrated the durability of this repair at 66 months with resolution of the false lumen.[10]

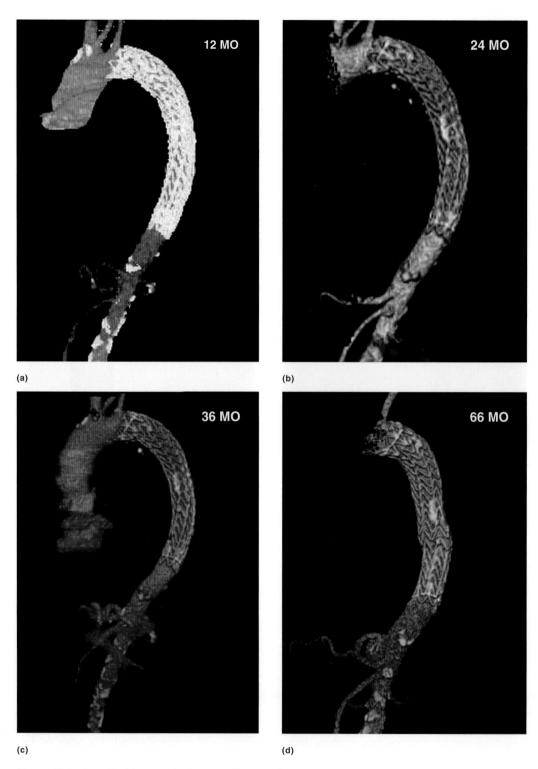

(a)

(b)

(c)

(d)

Figures 14-5 a, b, c, d Serial computerized tomographic scans of a treated type B dissection at 12, 24, 36, and 66 months post endograft placement. Note: The residual distal false lumen that was present at initial repair (0 months) has resolved by 12 months.

A promising therapy for aortic dissections is the Cook Dissection System. This system consists of a covered proximal Zenith TX2 thoracic stent graft and a distal component composed of open bare-metal Z-stents, figure 14-6. The open Z-stents exert minimal outward radial force to allow gradual apposition of the true and false lumens. Also the open Z-stents can be placed over the ostia of the renal and mesenteric arteries. Some surgeons have described this system as the "petticoat graft" based upon its appearance.

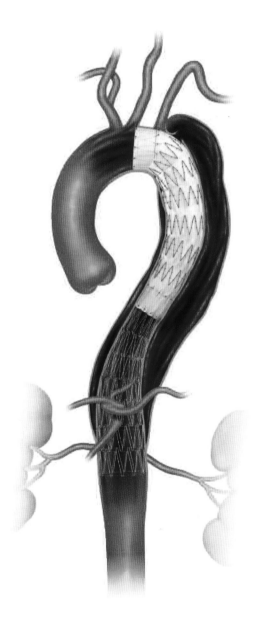

Figure 14-6 Cook Aortic Dissection System with proximal TX2 component and open stents distally. Illustration courtesy of Cook Medical, Bloomington, In.

REFERENCES

1. Tefera G, Archer CW, Hoch JR, et al. Effectiveness of Intensive Medical Therapy in Type B Aortic Dissection: A Single Center Experience. *Journal of Vascular Surgery.* 2007; 45 (6): 114.
2. Tsai T, Fattori R, Santi T, et al. Long-Term Survival in Patient Presenting with Type B Acute Aortic Dissections. Insights from the International Registry of Acute Aortic Dissection. *Circulation.* 2006; 114: 2226-2231.
3. Hagan PG, Nienaben CA, Isselbacher EM, et al. The International Registry of Acute Aortic Dissection: New Insights Into an Old Disease. *JAMA.* 2000 Feb. 16; 283 (7): 897-903.
4. Doroghazi RM, Glaren EE, DeSanctis RW, et al. Long-Term Survival of Patients with Treated Aortic Dissection. *Journal of American Collegiate Cardiology.* 1984; 3: 1026-1034.
5. Tsai TT, Evangelista A, Neinaber CA, et al. International Registry of Acute Aortic Dissection. Partial Thrombosis of the False Lumen in Patients with Acute Type B Aortic Dissections. *New England Journal of Medicine.* 2007 July 26; 357: 349-359.
6. Bernard Y, Zimmerman H, Chocron S, et al. False Lumen Patency is a Prediction of Late Outcome in Aortic Dissection. *American Journal of Cardiology.* 2001 June 15; 87 (12): 1378-1382.
7. Eggebrecht H, Nienaben C, Neuhauser M, et al. Endovascular Stent-Graft Placement in Aortic Dissection: A Meta-Analysis. *European Heart Journal.* 2006; 27: 489-498.
8. Nienaber C. INSTEAD Trial Preliminary Results. *Vascular.* 2006; 19 (Supplement 1).
9. Stevens SL, Farber MA, eds. *Thoracic Endovascular Aorta.* Knoxville, TN: Tennessee Valley Publishing; 2008.
10. Mitchell RO, Rogers AG, Earle GF, Imam M. Endograft Repair of Type B Aortic Dissection with Three-Year Follow-Up. *Journal of Kentucky Medical Association.* 2009; 107 (8): 291-293.

CHAPTER 15

Repair of a Residual Type A Dissection with Debranching and Antegrade Thoracic Endograft Delivery in a Single-Stage Procedure

Aneurysms and dissections of the transverse thoracic aorta have been associated with a high operative mortality. Open surgical replacement of the transverse arch has a mortality reported at 6%-31%.[1-4]

The elephant trunk technique described by Borst in 1983 allowed for a two-stage repair of extensive arch aneurysms that extend into the descending thoracic aorta.[5] The conventional elephant trunk technique became a recognized standard treatment modality for these extensive aneurysms in the 1980s thru 1990s. However, the elephant trunk procedure has some limitations. The larger reported series demonstrate a mortality of 2%-12% from stage 1 and a mortality of 3.9%-9.6% for stage 2.[6-8] In addition, there is a significant attrition between the two stages. A recent report indicates a 16% interval death rate between stages one and two of the elephant trunk procedure.[3]

Recently, as in the patient to be presented, hybrid procedures utilizing endografts and custom Dacron trifurcated branch grafts for arch revascularization have demonstrated a low operative mortality.[9-13] Although, the long-term durability of these repairs is yet unknown; the combination of new custom graft configurations with single stage endografts may eventually relegate the classical elephant trunk procedure to one of historical interest only.

There are rare reports of total endovascular arch repair with endografts and extra thoracic bypass.[13, 14] These repairs involve the use of double-barrel, parallel, or chimney grafts within the thoracic aorta. These techniques are discussed further in Chapter 12.

CASE SCENARIO:
Single-Stage Repair of
Aortic Dissection with Antegrade
ELG delivery

Three years previously, the patient presented with an extensive Stanford Type A dissection involving a disrupted aortic valve with extension into the infrarenal abdominal aorta. He underwent emergent aortic valve replacement, replacement of the ascending aorta, and bypass of two coronary arteries with saphenous vein grafts. Approximately 3 years following that procedure, surveillance CT scan demonstrated aneurysmal dilation in the residual dissection and the patient was referred to me for surgical consideration. The base of the innominate artery itself was enlarged to 4 cm and the aorta distal to the left subclavian artery was 7.4 cm, figure 15-1. The axial view is in figure 15-2. The illustration, figure 15-3, demonstrated the prior surgical repair and the enlarging dissection with a bovine arch anatomy. The dissection was repaired in a single-stage operation by using a combination of hypothermic circulatory arrest, cerebral debranching, repair of the aorta with a hand-sutured custom collar Siena graft, and antegrade delivery of a thoracic endograft.

The procedure was begun by placing bilat-

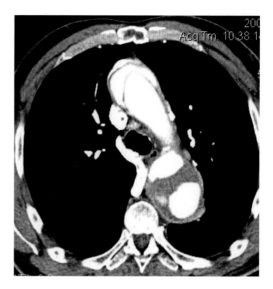

Figure 15-2 Computerized tomogram, axial view of aortic dissection.

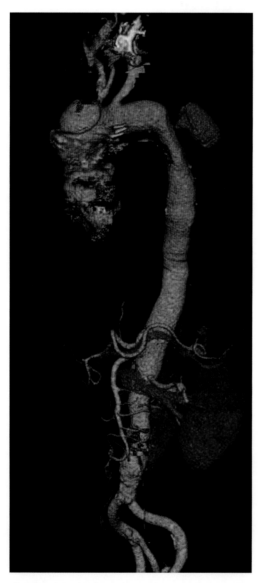

Figure 15-1 Computerized tomographic angiogram demonstrating aneurysmal dissection at innominate artery and distal to left subclavian artery.

eral radial artery catheters. The right axillary artery was cannulated with a 14-Fr cannula for right axillary and right atrial cardiopulmonary bypass. No aortic cross clamping was employed. After electroencephalographic silence was achieved, the transverse aortic arch was opened and the distal end of the Siena collar graft was placed in the true lumen of the distal aorta to extend for 6-8 cm. The collar was sutured to the open end of the transverse arch. The collar of the graft compensates for size disparities in the distal aorta.

Cerebral perfusion via the right axillary artery was maintained at a rate of 5-8 ml/kg/min with an inflow temperature of 16 degrees Celsius. Cerebral blood flow was monitored by the Somanetics System and EEG silence was maintained. The left subclavian artery was transected from the aortic arch and sutured in end-to-end fashion to one limb of a bifurcated graft. Cerebral perfusion was discontinued and the other end of the bifurcated graft was sutured in end-to-end fashion to the innominate artery. Note this patient had a bovine arch configuration and therefore a trifurcated graft to individually supply the left carotid artery was not needed. A trifurcated Dacron graft was

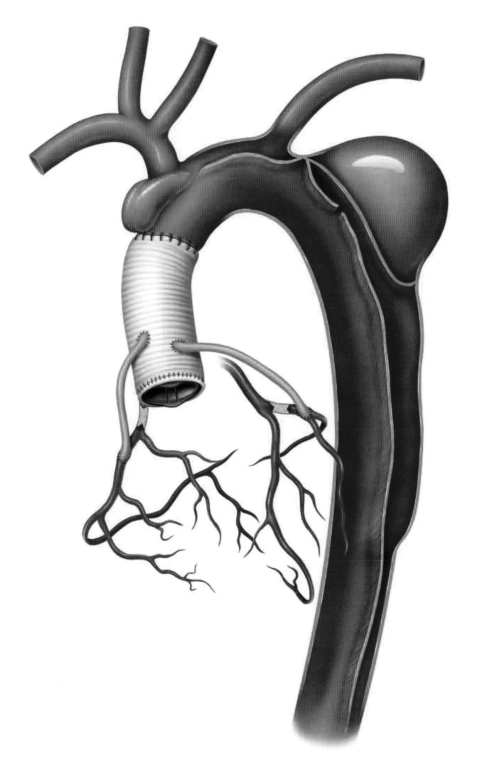

Figure 15-3 Illustration of previous surgery for Type A dissection and preoperative status for current surgery.

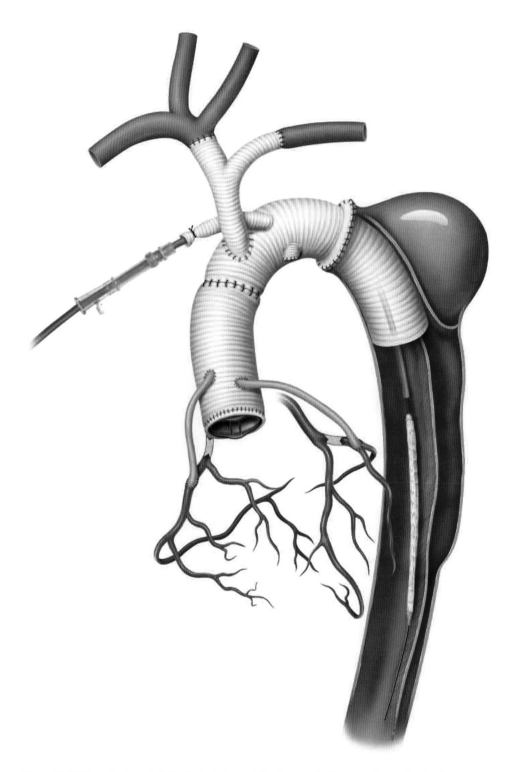

Figure 15-4 Delivery of antegrade ELG prior to deployment. The Siena graft will serve as the proximal landing zone.

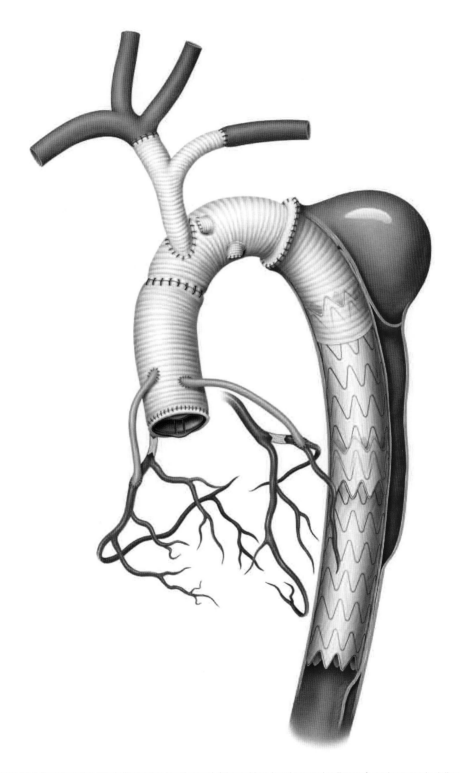

Figure 15-5 Postoperative repair illustrating head vessel debranching, hand-sutured collar-graft, and antegrade delivered thoracic endograft within the collar graft.

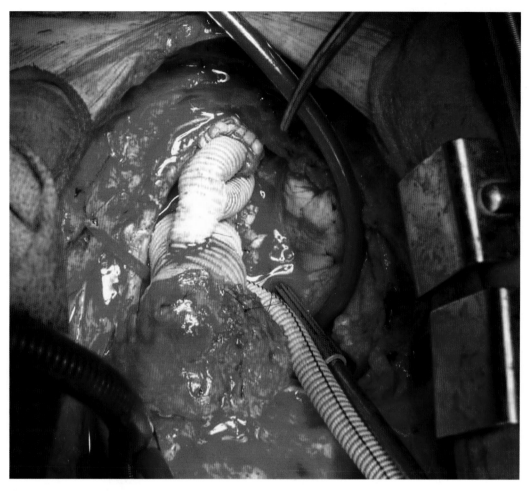

Figure 15-6 Intraoperative photograph of branch graft to head vessels.

modified on the back table prior to the start of the procedure to create a bifurcated graft. The cerebral circulatory arrest time was eight minutes.

As cerebral perfusion was resumed via the proximal end of the bifurcated graft, the proximal end of the Siena graft was sutured to the Dacron graft placed 3 years prior. Next, the proximal portion of the bifurcated graft was sutured to the side of the Siena graft. The thoracic endograft was deployed antegrade via the lateral sidearm, figure 15-4, of the graft as the patient was rewarmed by an arterial inflow cannula in the medial sidearm. The proximal landing zone

for the thoracic endograft is the distal end of the collared graft, figure 15-5.

The intraoperative photos of the head vessel grafts are seen in figure 15-6. The intraoperative arteriogram is seen in figure 15-7. The patient was extubated within one day of surgery and had no neurologic deficits. Computerized tomography 48 hours post operative demonstrates no evidence of endoleak, correction of the dissection throughout the descending thoracic aorta, and no compromise of blood flow to the carotid or subclavian arteries, figure 15-8. Follow-up CT angiogram eight months following repair demonstrated

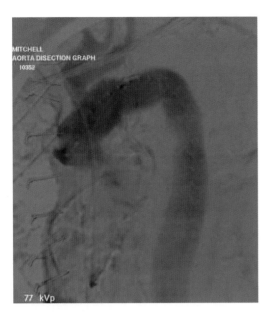

Figure 15-7 Intraoperative arteriogram of completed repair. Note: no endoleaks, resolution of aneurysmal segments, and no compromise of flow to the arch vessels.

near total resolution of the false lumen in the infrarenal aorta. The patient is doing well nearly two years postoperatively.

CASE DISCUSSION

It is common for patients with extensive type A dissections to return at a later time for correction of the transverse arch component secondary to enlargement. It is now my opinion, that in all but the most frail patients, the transverse arch should be corrected at the time of the initial type A dissection repair. If the transverse arch is involved with the dissection, it is easier to correct at the first operation instead of at reoperation. Whereas the aortic tissue may be friable, the great vessels are often able to hold sutures of the bifurcated or trifurcated Dacron graft. Additionally, if the original correction employs a collared-graft with the trunk extending into the distal true lumen, the residual dissection in the descending aorta can be addressed later with an endovascular approach. In short, I believe type A dissections that extend thru the transverse and

descending aorta should be thought of and treated as aneurysms rather than dissections and simply resuspending the aortic valve and placing a tube graft to the base of the innominate artery is inadequate for most patients.

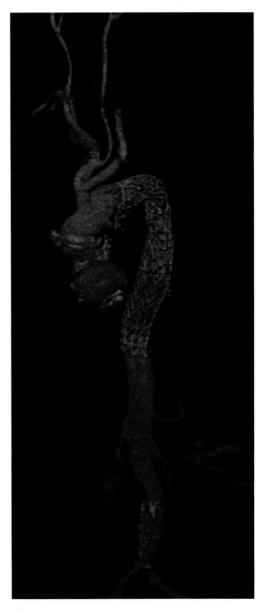

Figure 15-8 Computerized tomographic angiograms postoperative. Note that the collared-graft and the bifurcated branch graft do not appear "white" as they contain no metal as do the endograft.

Another option with this patient would be consideration of the E-vita graft (JOTEC, Hechingen, Ger.). This graft consists of a polyester tube affixed to a stent on one end and unstented polyester on the other end. The stented portion can be placed into the true lumen of the proximal descending thoracic aorta under direct vision or over a guidewire previously delivered retrograde under IVUS guidance to ensure true lumen placement. The unstented polyester end can accept great vessels as an island patch or be sutured to a trifurcated graft which can inturn be anastomosed to the great vessels individually. Because the stented portion of the graft is "fixed" with the proximal descending thoracic aorta, the technique is known as the "frozen elephant trunk".[15-17] A photograph of the E-vita graft can be seen in Chapter 23.

COMMENTARY

(Edward B. Diethrich, Phoenix, AZ) This chapter is of special interest to me since our original description of the antegrade approach for endoluminal graft deployment. However, while the technique is important and Dr. Mitchell's case presentation is extremely well done, his most important contribution in this chapter relates to the opening paragraph of the "case discussion" in which he opines "that in all but the most frail patients, the transverse arch should be corrected at the time of the initial type A dissection". That represents forward thinking and the current data are substantiating a similar position. It is projected that greater than 25% of patients left with only correction of the ascending aorta in type I (A) dissection will require further interventional treatment. I believe that number is considerably below the actual since many of these patients are lost to follow-up or die suddenly without treatment. It is perspectives like this that add immensely to our vascular future.

REFERENCES

1. Cooley DA, Goloma, Frazier OH. Single-Clamp Technique For Aneurysms of the Descending Thoracic Aorta: Report of 132 Consecutive Cases. *European Journal of Cardiothoracic Surgery.* 2000; 18 (2): 162-167.

2. Stone OH, Brewster DC, Kuolek CJ, et al. Stent-Graft versus Open Surgical Repair of the Thoracic Aorta: Midterm Results. *Journal of Vascular Surgery.* 2006; 44 (6): 1188.

3. Estrera A, Miller III CC, Chen EP, et al. Descending Thoracic Aortic Aneurysm Repair: 12-Year Experience Using Distal Aortic Perfusion and Cerebrospinal Fluid Drainage. *Annals of Thoracic Surgery.* 2005; 80 (40): 1290.

4. Verdant A, Cossette R, Page A, et al. Aneurysms of the Descending Thoracic Aorta: Three Hundred Sixty-Six Consecutive Cases Resected Without Paraplegia. *Journal of Vascular Surgery.* 1995; 21 (3): 385.

5. Borst HG, Walterbusch G, Schaps D. Extensive Aortic Replacement Using "Elephant Trunk" Prosthesis. *Thoracic Cardiovascular Surgery.* 1983; 31 (1): 37-40.

6. Safi HJ, Miller III CC, Estrera AL, Villa MA, et al. Optimization of Aortic Arch Replacement: Two-Stage Approach. *Annals of Thoracic Surgery.* 2007; 83 (2): 815-818.

7. Lemaire SA, Carter SA, Coselli JS. The Elephant Trunk Technique For Staged Repair of the Entire Thoracic Aorta. *Annals of Thoracic Surgery.* 2006; 81 (5): 1561-1569.

8. Suensson LG, Kim KH, Blackstone EH, et al. Elephant Trunk Procedure: Newer Indications and Uses. *Annals of Thoracic Surgery.* 2004; 78 (1): 109-116.

9. Hughes GC, Nienaber JJ, Bush EL, et al. Use of Custom Dacron Branch Grafts for "Hybrid" Aortic Debranching During Endovascular Repair of Thoracic and Thoracoabdominal Aortic Aneurysms. *Journal of Thoracic and Cardiovascular Surgery.* 2008; 136: 21-8.

10. Diethrich EB, Ghazoul M, Wheatley III GH, et al. Great Vessel Transposition for Antegrade Delivery of the TAG Endoprosthesis in the Proximal Aortic Arch. *Journal of Endovascular Therapy.* 2005; 582-587.

11. Mitchell RO, Rogers AG, Earle GF, Imam M. Hybrid Endovascular Repair of Thoracic Aortic Aneurysms By Debranching and the Creation of Landing Zone-Zero. *Journal of Kentucky Medical Association.* 2009; 107: 438-441.

12. Diethrich EB, Ramaiah VG, Kpodonu J, Rodriguez-Lopez JA. *Endovascular and Hybrid Management of the Thoracic Aorta.* Hoboken, NJ: Wiley-Blackwell Publishing; 2008.

13. Chuter TAM and Schneider DB. Endovascular Repair of the Aortic Arch. *Perspectives in Vascular Surgery and Endovascular Therapy.* 2007; 19 (2): 188-192.

14. Baldwin ZK, Chuter TAM, Hiramoto JS, et al. Double-Barrel Technique for Preservation of Aortic Arch Branches During Thoracic Endovascular Aortic Repair. *Annals of Vascular Surgery.* 2008; 22: 703-709.

15. Karck M, Chavan A, Hagel C, et al. The Frozen Elephant Trunk Technique: A New Treatment for Thoracic Aortic Aneurysms. *Journal of Thoracic Cardiovascular Surgery.* 2003; 125: 1550-1553.

16. Jsui A, Veda Y, Watanabe T, et al. Clinical Results of Implantation of an Endovascular Covered Stent-Graft Via Midsternotomy for Distal Aortic Arch Aneurysm. *Cardiovascular Surgery.* 2000; 8 (7): 545-549.

17. Karck M. and Kamiya H. Progress of the Treatment for Extended Aortic Aneurysms; Is the Frozen Elephant Trunk Technique the Next Standard in the Treatment of Complex Aortic Disease Including the Arch? *European Journal of Cardiothoracic Surgery.* 2008; 33: 1007-1013.

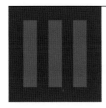

SECTION III

Other Cardiovascular Pathology

CHAPTER 16

Alternative Arterial Access Routes for Endograft Delivery and Associated Complications

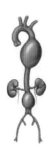

The fault is not in our stars, but in ourselves.
– William Shakespeare, Julius Caesar (I.ii.140-141)

Obtaining arterial access for both endovascular aortic aneurysm repair (EVAR) and thoracic endovascular aortic aneurysm repair (TEVAR) is a critical component of the procedure. This is especially true of TEVAR, as larger access sheaths are required. Sheath-related iliac artery dissections or disruptions are one of the most common causes of intraoperative death. Overall, vascular complications account for nearly 20% of the major adverse events during TEVAR. In addition, as many as 20% of the patients will require an arterial conduit or alternative arterial access site for

TEVAR access.[1-7] Figure 16-1 demonstrates a 4-Fr sheath, which can be used for diagnostic coronary imaging and the 18-Fr sheath often used for EVAR. The 24-Fr sheaths are often required for TEVAR. An often confusing issue is that the inner dilators are sized in the French system based upon their outer diameter. Whereas the actual sheaths are sized upon the French system based on their inner diameter. Obviously, it is the outer diameter of the sheath that produces the hole of a corresponding size in a given artery.

Careful preoperative case planning with at-

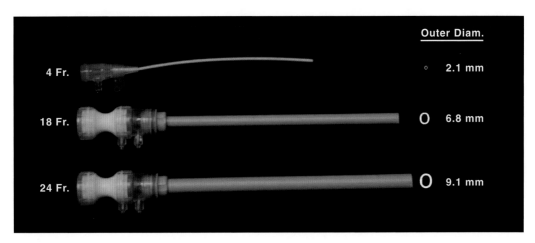

Figure 16-1 Photograph to compare arterial access sheaths and outer diameter in millimeters.

tention to femoral artery and iliac artery diameters as determined by axial computerized tomography is necessary to avoid these complications. TEVAR in women is potentially problematic for two reasons. First, women tend to have smaller access arteries than men. Secondly, women comprise a relatively higher proportion of patients with thoracic aneurysms as compared to patients with abdominal aneurysms (ratio of male-female TAA 60:40; ratio male-female AAA 80:20).

In addition to computerized tomographic measurements of arterial diameter, the surgeon's judgment regarding arterial calcification and tortuosity is critical. Some arteries that are deemed of adequate size by CT-scan, may be too calcified or too torturous to accommodate a sheath in standard fashion. The following chapter will discuss arterial access adjuncts and alternatives including: angioplasty, endoconduits, iliac conduits, semi-bareback delivery, side-branch delivery, and antegrade delivery. Finally, the chapter will conclude with the "peel-away sheath" technique for endovascular repair of iliac disruption.

ANGIOPLASTY AND ENDOCONDUITS

The simplest adjunct for arterial access is balloon angioplasty. An 8 mm angioplasty balloon will correct focal iliac stenosis and allow for passage of 16 or 18 French sheath needed for EVAR access. However, a discreet area of stenosis flanked by normal artery is not the usual case scenario. More commonly diffuse iliac disease is present. In addition, extensively calcified iliac arteries may be prone to dissect with aggressive angioplasty. A covered stent-graft (endoconduit) will protect against exsanguination from an iliac artery dissection. This technique of angioplasty with graft coverage has been called "cracking and paving".[8] I prefer a 9 mm Viabahn covered stent graft. This graft can tolerate aggressive angioplasty with little concern for iliac artery bleeding. In addition, the smooth inner lining of a 9 mm Viabahn graft will easily accommodate a 20-Fr sheath. A potential concern during sheathless or "bareback" delivery of the GORE Excluder or TAG endograft is premature inadvertent deployment if the release string becomes entangled

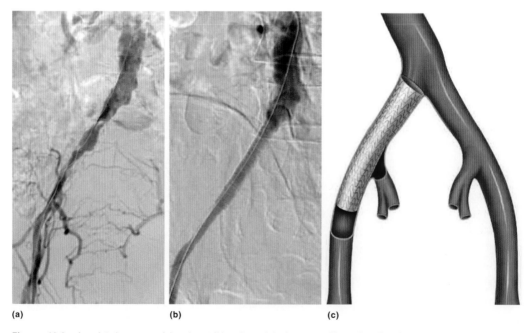

(a) (b) (c)

Figures 16-2 a, b, c Arteriogram pre (a) and post (b) endoconduit placement. Illustration of endoconduit in the iliac artery (c).

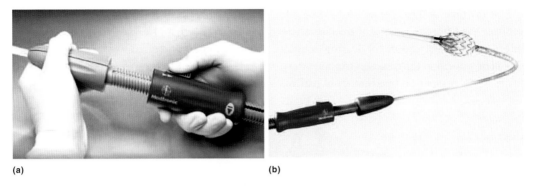

(a)   (b)

Figures 16-3 a, b Medtronic delivery sheath and contained endograft. Photo courtesy Medtronic corporation.

on a calcified area of the arterial wall. The smooth inner lining of a Viabahn endoconduit mitigates against this premature deployment. Figures 16-2 a, b, c demonstrate and illustrate iliac arterial stenosis corrected with an endoconduit for subsequent large sheath and endograft access. A potential disadvantage of the covered endoconduit is loss of the internal iliac artery. If the contralateral internal iliac artery is occluded the risk of gluteal claudication and/or colon ischemia must be weighed and other access strategies considered.

The Talent abdominal endograft (Medtronic Corporation, Santa Rosa, CA) utilizes a self-contained system with a combined endograft within the delivery sheath, figures 16-3a and 3b. The delivery device has a hydrophilic coating and tapered end. When exposed to water/saline it has an extremely low frictional coefficient, for ease of insertion.

BALLOON - EXPANDABLE SHEATHS

A promising new technology is the balloon-expandable sheath. SoloPath (Onset Medical Corp., Irvine, CA) is a sheath that enters the femoral artery with an outer diameter of 13.5-Fr. The sheath is supplied with an inner balloon that dilates the sheath to an outer diameter of 21-Fr. The sheath then serves as an endoconduit for ELG or TAVI delivery. The sheath then passively collapses at removal.

ILIAC ARTERY CONDUIT

The most common method for managing difficult vascular access is by construction of iliac artery conduits. This may be required in 20% of the patients undergoing TEVAR. In this technique, a flank incision will allow retroperitoneal access to the common iliac artery. An 8mm or 10 mm Dacron graft can be sutured to the common iliac artery and the delivery sheath can be deployed via that open end of the Dacron graft, figure 16-4a. An umbilical tape tied around the Dacron will prevent back bleeding. Alternatively, the sheath can be placed into the side of the Dacron graft. The left common iliac artery should be used for conduit placement, as exposure is generally easier. Most diseased iliac arteries seem to match an 8 mm rather than 10 mm graft. A 22- Fr sheath will pass through an 8 mm Dacron conduit despite the fact that the outer diameter of a 22-Fr sheath is generally about 8.2 mm. If a 24-Fr sheath is required a 10 mm conduit should be used. The conduit should not be placed on the external iliac artery, but rather on the common iliac artery midway between the aortic bifurcation and internal iliac origin. If the conduit is placed on the external iliac artery and a dissection/disruption occurs during sheath removal, back-bleeding from the internal iliac artery may be problematic. Disruptions generally occur at the external/internal iliac artery bifurcation.

At the time of sheath removal, a retrograde contrast hand injection can confirm iliac artery integrity. The distal end of the Dacron conduit should be sutured to the common femoral artery, figure 16-4b. A significant percentage of patients will require re-intervention, and this conduit will serve as a future access site. It seems the intervening section of artery will thrombose over time; however, I have not seen other documented reports of this.

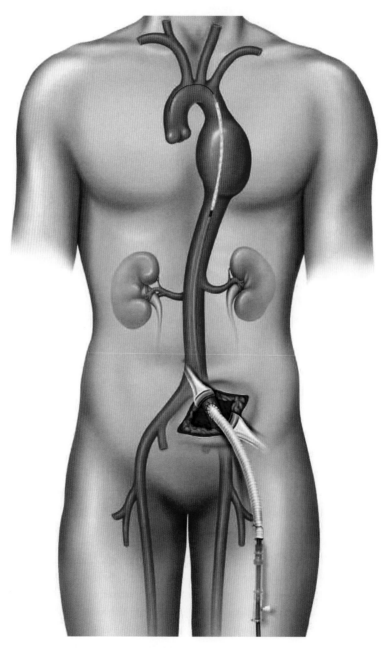

Figure 16-4a Sheath placement via Dacron iliac artery conduit.

BAREBACK AND SEMI-BAREBACK TECHNIQUE

Endografts such as the Excluder and TAG (W. L. Gore and Associates, Flagstaff, AZ) may be

delivered sheathless or "bareback." The absence of a sheath effectively reduces that needed diameter of the access vessel. The manufacturer specifically discourages this technique. Potential problems include an "unsmooth" delivery, which may cause

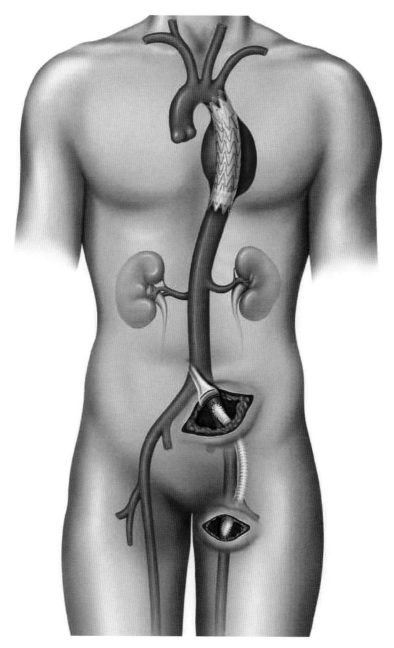

Figure 16-4b Thoracic ELG deployed and distal end of conduit sutured to femoral artery allows for future endovascular access.

premature deployment of the device and access site bleeding. The access site bleeding is usually the result of a previous failed attempt to pass a larger sheath and the resultant hole in the artery is larger than the bareback device.

The semi-bareback technique will minimize access site bleeding. Often the introducer and sheath will pass a few centimeters into the artery but no further. If preoperative measurements or intravascular ultrasound indicate the bareback

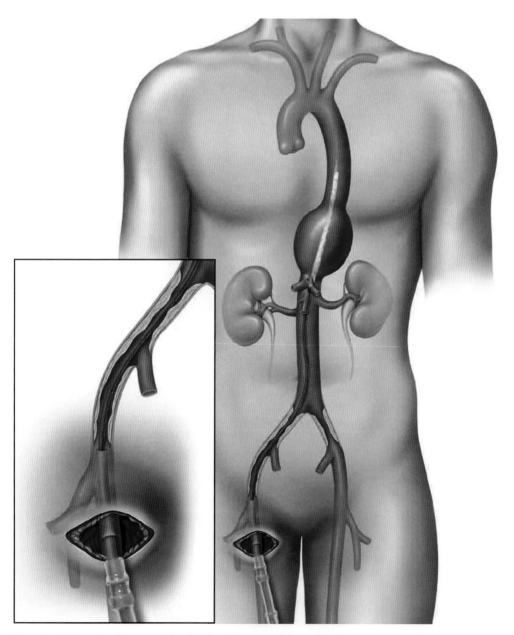

Figure 16-5 Illustration of shortened-sheath and semi-bareback delivery of a thoracic endograft. Only 2 cm of "cut-off" sheath enters artery for hemostatic control. The graft is delivered "bareback" through the narrowed artery.

device could traverse the artery, then the sheath can be cut to a maximum length of 2 to 4 cm and replaced over the introducer. This shortened-sheath is placed a few centimeters into the common femoral artery. The endograft device is then delivered initially through the sheath and then bareback into final position, figure 16-5. This will significantly minimize access site bleeding and provide an element of control for the use of buddy wires or pigtail catheters.

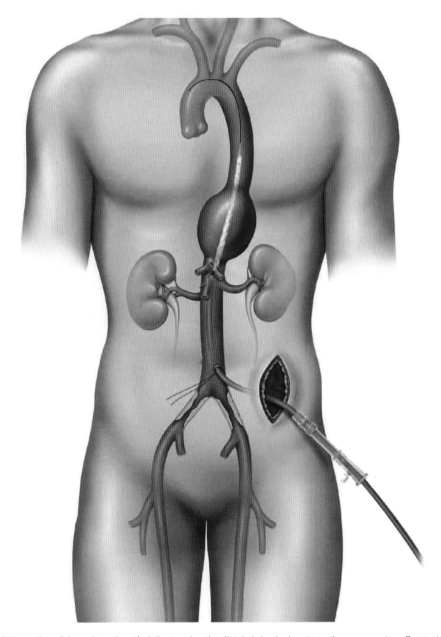

Figure 16-6 Illustration of thoracic endograft delivery using the distal abdominal aorta as the access artery. Purse-string sutures used instead of a conduit.

USE OF THE DISTAL ABDOMINAL AORTA FOR TEVAR ACCESS

In the event the iliac system cannot accommodate the large sheaths needed for TEVAR, Dacron conduits may be sutured to the distal abdominal aorta. Alternatively, purse-string sutures may be placed in the abdominal aorta. The following case scenario describes a patient who underwent direct distal abdominal aortic cannulation for TEVAR access.

CASE SCENARIO:
Direct Infrarenal Abdominal Aortic Cannulation for TEVAR

The patient is a 79-year-old man with a 6.8 cm aneurysm involving the distal thoracic aorta and proximal abdominal aorta extending to a few centimeters above the celiac artery. Preoperative computerized tomographic measurements indicated the iliac arteries were not large enough to accommodate the necessary 22-Fr sheath. The iliac arteries were also too small for a sutured iliac conduit to be effective. In this case the distal abdominal aorta was exposed using a retroperitoneal approach via a left flank incision. The distal aorta was extensively calcified and it seemed difficult to obtain adequate control in order to suture a Dacron conduit directly to the aorta. I also had concerns that a side-biting clamp could cause distal plaque embolization. Polypropylene purse-string sutures were placed on the distal abdominal aorta for subsequent direct wire and sheath cannulation, figure 16-6. Postoperative computerized tomographic angiogram demonstrates exclusion of the aneurysm with no endoleak 60 months post-procedure. Note the calcified and small iliac arteries, figure 16-7.

A few days following discharge from the hospital, this patient returned with a relatively sudden onset of lower extremity paresis. Emergent CT scan confirmed no endograft migration or other changes from his postoperative scan. It was noted, however, that the patient's systolic blood pressure was approximately 90 mmHg. A Swan-

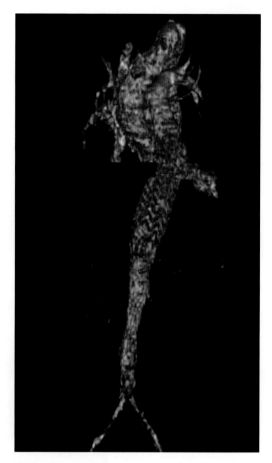

Figure 16-7 Postoperative computerized tomographic angiogram 60 months post-procedure demonstrating thoracic endograft placed via abdominal aortic access. Note calcified and small iliac arteries, which prevented standard femoral graft delivery.

Ganz catheter was placed to monitor fluid resuscitation in this patient with know cardiac dysfunction. In addition, a spinal drain was placed and pressure agents used to maintain a systolic blood pressure of 140 mmHg. Within 8-10 hours of presentation to the hospital, the patient began to have return of neurologic function. At the time of his second hospital discharge he was ambulatory and had regained full neurologic function. This patient was managed early in my experience with thoracic endografts. Current practice is to slowly restart or stagger the start of the patient's home antihypertensive medications to avoid any potential hypotension in the early postoperative period.

This is especially true with endograft coverage of upper abdominal aorta or with coverage of long segments of the thoracoabdominal aorta. This patient is currently 85 years of age and doing well. However, his renal insufficiency precludes a CT scan with contrast.

ABDOMINAL AORTA REPLACEMENT FOR TEVAR ACCESS

The patient is a 69-year-old woman with a 5.4 cm infrarenal abdominal aortic aneurysm and a 6.3 cm thoracic aorta aneurysm. The intervening mesore-

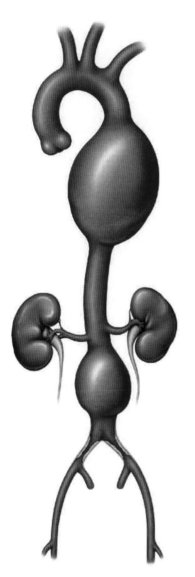

Figure 16-8 Illustration of separate thoracic and abdominal aortic aneurysms with small and calcified iliac arteries.

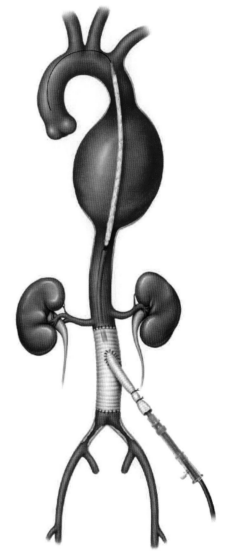

Figure 16-9 Illustration of thoracic endograft delivered via a side-branch of a hand-sutured abdominal graft at time of laparotomy.

nal aorta was not aneurysmal. The iliac arteries were significantly calcified and small. Preoperative measurements indicated the iliac arteries would not accommodate the 24-Fr sheath needed for thoracic endograft delivery, as illustrated in figure 16-8. In this patient, the abdominal aorta was repaired by laparotomy and open aneurysmorraphy using a hand-sutured Dacron tube graft. This particular Dacron tube graft is supplied by the

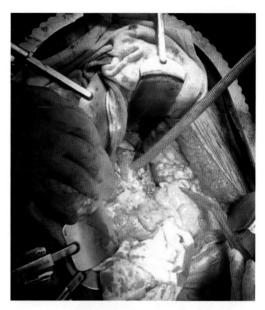

Figure 16-11 Intraoperative photograph. Thoracic endograft delivered via side-branch of Dacron tube graft at time of open infrarenal aortic aneurysm repair.

manufacturer with a 10 mm Dacron side arm, which would be used to deliver the thoracic endograft, figure 16-9. The intraoperative photograph, figure 16-11 shows the 10 mm side arm extending from the Dacron tube graft at time of laparotomy. Figure 16-10 illustrates the completed procedure. Computerized tomographic angiogram at one-year follow-up is seen in figure 16-12. The use of an abdominal aortic graft for TEVAR access has been reported by other authors.[9-11]

Although this patient is progressing satisfactory nearly six years post procedure, is it now well-established that there is an increased risk of paralysis during TEVAR if a patient has had a previous open abdominal aortic aneurysm repair.[12, 13] It would be reasonable to assume that concomitant abdominal aneurysm repair and TEVAR would also have an increased risk of paralysis; however, I am unaware of data specifically addressing this relatively unusual procedure.

The field of endovascular surgery is advancing and expanding rapidly. Similarly, this patient might be managed differently in my current practice. Specifically, a spinal drain would certainly

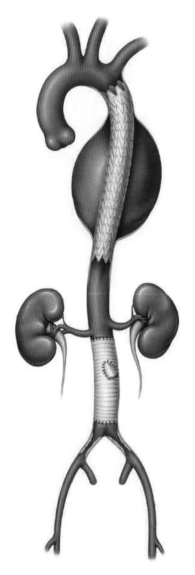

Figure 16-10 Illustration of completed repair: Open abdominal aortic aneurysmorraphy and concomitant thoracic endovascular aortic aneurysm repair (TEVAR).

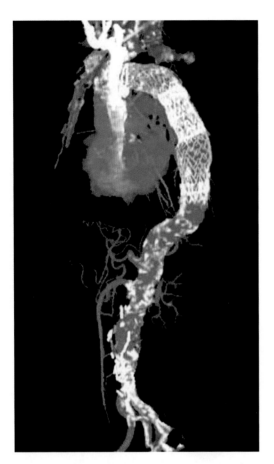

Figure 16-12 Computerized tomographic angiogram after open abdominal aneurysmorraphy and thoracic aortic aneurysm endografting.

be used in the case of concomitant TEVAR and open abdominal aneurysm repair. Spinal drainage was not performed during this patient's surgery six years prior. Additionally, more thought may have been given regarding open repair of the abdominal aneurysm with a bifurcated Dacron graft. The femoral limbs could provide access for future endovascular intervention in this patient with relatively small native iliac arteries. Even the concept of the concomitant TEVAR and open abdominal aneurysmorraphy may have yielded to a "staged" approach with TEVAR access via the femoral limb of the abdominal graft weeks or even months later. I had to weigh these considerations against the possibility of a graft infection secondary to a potential infected groin incision associated with the

bifurcated aortic grafts. It is only through critically and objectively evaluating our past work that we insure the best care for our patients in the future.

ANTEGRADE ENDOGRAFT DELIVERY

Thoracic endografts can be delivered antegrade via a conduit in the ascending aortic arch.[6, 7, 14] This technique is discussed in more detail in Chapter 15. Antegrade delivery is utilized either because the iliac arteries are too small to accommodate the large TEVAR sheaths or more commonly because the surgeon is already working in the open chest for a concomitant procedure.

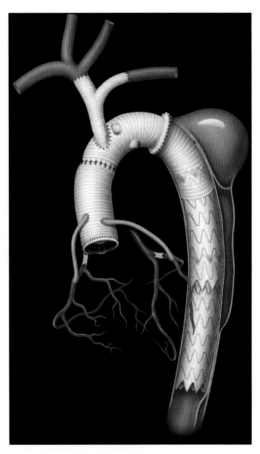

Figure 16-13 Illustration of antegrade thoracic endograft via a customized collared plexus graft, described further in Chapter 15.

CASE SCENARIO:
Antegrade Endograft Delivery

Three years prior, the patient had presented with an extensive Stanford Type-A aortic dissection extending from the avulsed aortic valve to below the renal arteries. I had repaired his ascending aorta using a Dacron graft, replaced his aortic valve, which I was unable to resuspend, and bypassed two coronary arteries with reverse saphenous vein grafts. In the three years since the surgery, the dissection in the transverse and proximal descending thoracic aorta had become aneurysmal with a diameter of 7 cm. This was repaired via reoperative median sternotomy, replacement of the transverse aortic arch with a collared Siena graft

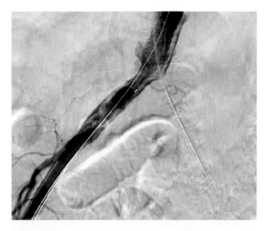

Figure 16-14 Hand injection of contrast into right femoral sheath with intimal tear in right iliac artery. Note unusual contrast configuration and bulbous shape of right iliac artery just distal to graft limb.

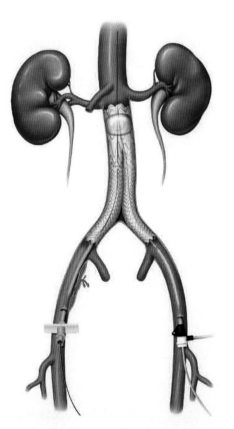

Figure 16-15a Right iliac artery dissection extending to sheath entry site. Aortic occlusion balloon placed via left femoral sheath for control of bleeding. Peel-away sheath placed over right-sided wire through original sheath entry site.

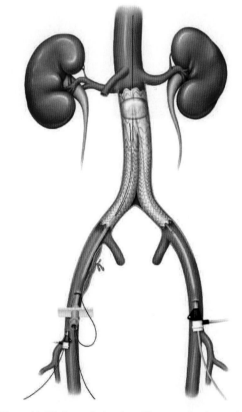

Figure 16-15b Second wire placed in artery distal to peel-away sheath and wire brought out of peel-away sheath's entry site and placed into peel-away sheath as a buddy-wire. The peel-away sheath and original wire are removed.

extending as a stage-I elephant trunk, head vessel debranching, and concomitant antegrade thoracic endograft delivery via the side-arm of the Siena graft, figure 16-13. In this patient, antegrade delivery was convenient as the chest was already open. Additionally, antegrade delivery virtually eliminated the possibility of false-lumen deployment. Regardless of antegrade or retrograde delivery, the placement of a thoracic endograft in the hand-sutured trunk eliminated the need for the thoracotomy which would be required in the traditional stage-II of the elephant trunk procedure. This case illustrates another principle. In my opinion Type-A dissections that have a transverse arch component should be corrected at the time of the initial surgery. This should be done in all but the most frail and elderly patients. It seems that undoubtedly after a period of time, the dissection in the transverse arch does become problematic.

MANAGEMENT OF ILIAC ARTERY DISSECTION USING THE PEEL-AWAY SHEATH TECHNIQUE

Vascular complications account for 20% of the major adverse events during thoracic endografting. Specifically, iliac artery dissection or disruption is a leading cause of death during endovascular aneurysm repair. This is also showing itself to be a problem with TAVI transfemoral aortic valve replacement. The following

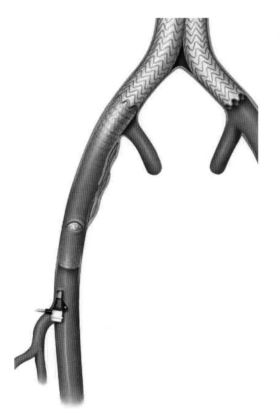

Figure 16-15c Viabahn graft is placed via new wire to extend from distal end of endograft and exclude both the dissection and the original sheath entry site.

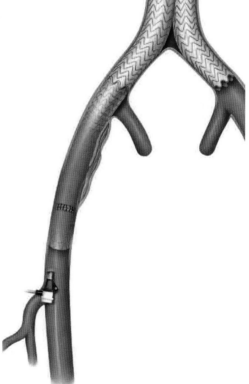

Figure 16-15d Closure of adventitia over exposed Viabahn graft.

case scenario discusses the successful endovascular management of an iliac artery dissection which occurred during EVAR.

CASE SCENARIO:
Iliac Dissection

The patient is a 79-year-old woman with an infrarenal abdominal aortic aneurysm. Preoperative case planning and computerized tomographic measurements had indicated the iliac arteries to be only marginally adequate to accommodate the necessary sheaths. Additionally, the left iliac system had undergone extensive bare metal stenting two years prior at another hospital.

Under general anesthesia, the femoral arteries were identified by cutdown. The right common femoral artery was cannulated high near the base of the inguinal ligament where it appeared to be a good quality vessel. A 0.035 inch guide wire was placed in the mid thoracic aorta using fluoroscopic visualization. The wire was changed to a stiff 0.035 inch wire followed by a 16-Fr introducer sheath. EVAR was carried out uneventfully using a bifurcated endograft. The completion aortogram demonstrated no evidence of endoleak; however a hand-held contrast injection through the right femoral sheath demonstrated a suspicious bulbous configuration of contrast in a subintimal flap at the distal end of the right graft limb, figure 16-14. Upon complete removal of the right femoral sheath, intima was noted to be protruding from the access site of the near pulseless right femoral artery. Wire access had been maintained and a Viabahn covered stent graft was used to correct the arterial injury. The following text and illustrations will describe what I call the "peel-away sheath technique" for repairing iliac artery dissections or injuries. This technique is especially useful in situations such as this where the dissection extends all the way to the sheath entry site.

First, and most importantly, never lose wire access as the femoral sheaths are removed. The wire is always the last device to be removed. A retrograde hand-injection of contrast through the

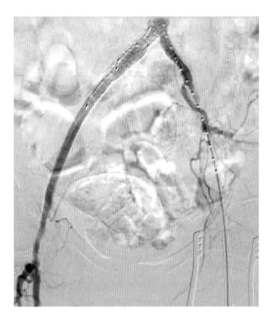

Figure 16-16 Intraoperative arteriogram demonstrating repair of right iliac artery dissection with covered Viabahn graft. Note preservation of profunda femoris artery.

sheath just before its removal will document artery integrity. Additionally, aortic occlusion balloons should always be available in the endo suite. An aortic occlusion balloon placed within the aortic graft via the contralateral sheath will eliminate a majority of bleeding. At the completion of the procedure, I tend to always remove the largest sheath first. The largest sheath is the most likely to cause an iliac dissection and the contralateral sheath can then be used to place the aortic occlusion balloon.

A long peel-away sheath, that is commonly used for inserting pacemaker leads or dialysis access catheters, is placed over the wire from the original sheath entry site, figure 16-15a. Peel-away sheaths (Tearaway Sheath - Galt Medical Corp., Garland, TX) come in lengths of 30 cm and will easily reach to the aortic bifurcation. The femoral artery is then accessed with a second 0.035 inch wire which enters the femoral artery 1-2 cm distal to the original access site. This second wire is brought out the original sheath entry hole beside of the peel-away sheath and then advanced through the peel-away sheath as a buddy wire into the aortic portion of the endograft, figure 16-15b. The first wire is removed, the sheath is peeled-apart and removed, and the new wire now traverses the original entry site and into the true lumen (endograft limb). The peel-away sheath guarantees that the second wire will be in the true lumen. An appropriately sized Viabahn covered graft is deployed over the second wire to connect the distal limb of the endograft and span/seal both the dissection and the original sheath entry site, figure 16-15c. The adventitia is closed over the visible Viabahn so that no graft remains exposed, figure 16-15d. Completion intraoperative arteriogram demonstrates the repaired artery with preservation of the profoundus femoral artery, figure 16-16.

COMMENTARY

(Dennis R. Gable, Plano, TX) Chapter 16 provides a nice overview of options available for patients that have difficult access when pursuing endovascular treatment. These options and techniques are commonly used in current day practice and allow for preserving treatment options through an endovascular modality rather than converting to an open surgery due to the inability to deliver the endovascular device. This chapter provides a nice outline of multiple different options both for thoracic and aortic devices.

REFERENCES

1. Bavaria JE, Appoo JJ, Makaroun MS, et al. Endovascular stent grafting versus open surgical repair of descending thoracic aortic aneurysm in low risk patients: A multicenter comparative trial. *J Thorac Cardiovasc Surg.* 2007; 133 (2): 369-377.

2. Farber MA. Complications of Endovascular Aortic Repair. *Texas Heart Institute Journal.* 2009; 36 (5): 444-445.

3. Makaroun MS., Dillavou ED, Wheatley GH, et al. Five-year results of endovascular treatment with the Gore TAG device compared with open repair of thoracic aortic aneurysms. *J Vasc Surg.* 2008; 47: 912-918.

4. Fairman RM, Criado F, Farber M, et al. Pivotal results of the Medtronic vascular Talent thoracic stent graft system: The VALOR trial. *J Vasc Surg.* 2008; 48: 546-554.

5. Matsumura JS, Lambria RP, Dake MD, et al. International controlled clinical trial of thoracic endovascular aneurysm repair with the Zenith TX2 endovascular graft: 1-year results. *J Vasc Surg.* 2008; 47 (2): 247-257.

6. Lumsden AB, Lin PH, Chen C, Parodi JC. *Advanced endovascular therapy of aortic disease.* Malden, MA: Blackwell Publishing; 2007.

7. Diethrich EB, Ramaiah VG, Pkodonu J, Rodriguez-Lopez JA. *Endovascular and hybrid management of the thoracic aorta.* Hoboken, NJ: Wiley-Blackwell Publishers; 2008.

8. Diethrich EB. "Cracking and Paving" A novel technique to delver a thoracic endograft despite ilio-femoral occlusive disease. *J Card Surg.* 2009; 24: 188-190.

9. Sugimoto I, Ohta T, Ishibashi H, et al. Simultaneous open and endoluminal repair of ruptured abdominal and thoracic aortic aneurysms: Report of a case. *Surg Today.* 2004; 24: 961-964.

10. Moon MR, Mitchell RS, Dake MD, et al. Simultaneous abdominal aortic replacement and thoracic stent-graft placement for multilevel aortic disease. *J Vasc Surg.* 1997; 25: 332-340.

11. Wolf YG, Zarins CK, Rubin GD, et al. Concomitant endovascular repair of descending thoracic and abdominal aortic aneurysm. *Circulation.* 2000; 102: e36.

12. Fatton R, Napoli G, Lavuto L, et al. Descending thoracic aortic diseases: Stent-graft repair. *Radiology.* 2003; 229 (1): 176-183.

13. Criado FJ, Clark NS. Barnatan MF. Stent graft repair in the aortic arch and descending thoracic aorta: A 4-year experience. *J Vasc Surg.* 2002; 36 (6): 1121-1128.

14. Diethrich EB, Ghazal M, Wheatley III GH, et al. Great vessel transposition for antegrade deliver o the TAG endoprosthesis in the proximal aortic arch. *J. Endovasc Ther.* 2005; 12: 583-587

CHAPTER 17

Endovascular Aortic Occlusive Repair (EVOR) with Bifurcated Endografts

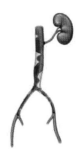

Atherosclerotic occlusive disease of the aortoiliac arteries is common and may be extremely disabling.[1,2] Symptoms may include thigh/buttock claudication, impotence, rest pain, and tissue loss. The gold-standard therapy for diffuse aortoiliac occlusive disease is the aortobifemoral bypass. This procedure yields patency rates of 86% to 94% at five years and 70% at 10 years. Advantages of the aortoiliac bypass include not only its excellent patency rates, but also its ability to treat "long-segment" diffuse disease or complete obstruction of the aortoiliac system. However, the aortobifemoral bypass is not without disadvantages. The invasiveness of the procedure is significant and complication rates of 30% and mortality rates of 2% to 5% have been reported.[3-8] Many elderly patients or patients with multiple co-morbidities are often not candidates for an operation of this magnitude. Even younger patients may expect a 5 to 7 day hospital stay and 8 to 12 weeks before returning to work. In addition, the bilateral groin incisions are a potential site of infection with subsequent infection of the underlying prosthetic graft.

Some patients with the so-called "hostile abdomen" from multiple previous abdominal surgeries or peritonitis are also poor candidates for aortobifemoral bypass grafting via the anterior laparotomy approach. Such patients may undergo a retroperitoneal approach using a flank incision.

There are also reports of avoiding the hostile abdomen to construct a thoracic aorta to bifemoral bypass.[9] Figure 17-1 illustrates a thoracic aorta to bifemoral bypass.

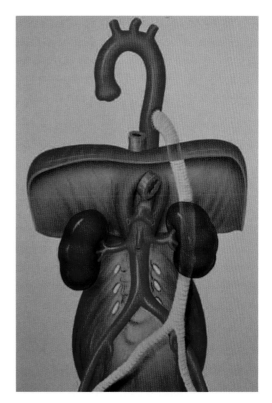

Figure 17-1 Illustration of thoracic aorta to bifemoral bypass.[9]

The femoral to femoral cross-over graft can treat unilateral iliac artery stenosis/occlusion and does not require an abdominal incision. However, patency rates are inferior to the aortobifemoral bypass and this technique cannot treat aortic occlusive disease or bilateral iliac disease.[10-12]

The axillary artery to bifemoral bypass is an alternative for the very elderly or patients with significant co-morbidities. This operation does not require an intracavitary body incision and has less likelihood of causing hemodynamic instability or fluid-shifts in such frail patients. However, groin incisions with underlying prosthetic graft material still pose an infection risk. In addition, the long-term patency of femorofemoral and axillofemoral grafts is poor with reported five year patency rates of only 45% to 65%.[13-16]

Percutaneous angioplasty and stenting of common iliac artery stenosis is appealing for a number of reasons. First, the procedure is relatively simply to perform and there is an initial technical success rate of 90-100% for focal common iliac artery stenosis. Secondly, the procedure is much less invasive than open surgical revascularization. Finally, the hospital length of stay is minimal and patients may theoretically return to work promptly.

However, despite the intuitive appeal of angioplasty and bare-metal stenting, this solution is far from perfect. Stenting of focal common iliac stenosis has a 20% failure rate at one year. Selective stenting of longer iliac lesions has been shown to have a patency rate of 50-80% at four years post stenting.[17-20] Even more problematic is diffuse atherosclerotic disease involving both the common and external iliac arterial systems. A meta-analysis of studies with angioplasty and stenting of con-comitant common and external iliac artery disease demonstrates a primary patency rate of only 70% at two years.[19] Subgroups of these patients with poor distal runoff have a primary patency rate after stent placement of only 30% at 12 months.[21,22] The poor results of catheter-based intervention in this subset has prompted the Transatlantic Inter-Soci-ety Consensus (T.A.S.C.) group to recommend open aortobifemoral bypass for qualified patients with T.A.S.C. Class C and D iliac disease.[23]

Failure of bare-metal stenting is multifactorial and related to: poor distal arterial runoff, multi or long segment iliac disease, and intimal hyperplasia. Intimal hyperplasia occurs in the region of the stented artery and immediately adjacent to the stented segment. The myointimal growth proliferates through the intersticies of the bare-metal stent and causes re-stenosis. The use of a stent with a fabric covering (endograft) would theoretically prevent intimal hyperplasia from causing re-stenosis as the fabric would serve as a mechanical barrier against cell ingrowth.

The use of covered stents (endografts) was reported in 1995 for the treatment of failed aortoiliofemoral reconstructions.[24] This report detailed the construction and use of "homemade" stent grafts to treat stenosis within native arteries or within the limbs of prosthetic bypass grafts. In all cases, 6 mm polytetrafluoroethylene grafts (PTFE) were hand-sutured into balloon-expand-able Palmaz stents and delivered to the remote target vessel via arterial cut-down. The follow-up results of this study were published in 1999.[25]

Between the years 2000 and 2005, reports from Europe and the United States described the use of commercially produced stent grafts to treat occlusive disease[26-29]: Hemobahn and Viabahn (W. L. Gore and Associates, Flagstaff, AZ), Wallgraft (Boston Scientific Corp, Boston, MA), and the iCAST stent graft (Atrium Medical Corp, Hudson, NH). The grafts used in all of these series were mono-grafts or tubular devices.

The first reported use of a bifurcated endoprosthesis to treat aortoiliac occlusive disease was in 2005.[30] This report described five patients with iliac artery stenosis or occlusive disease. Four patients underwent initial thrombolytic therapy and all underwent second-stage placement of a bifurcated Excluder endograft the following day. Technical (angiographic) success as well as improvement in ankle-brachial indices was achieved in all patients.

The below case scenario describes the use of a bifurcated endoprosthesis to treat a patient with aortoiliac occlusive disease in a "single-stage" procedure. I have termed the use of an endograft for endovascular aortic occlusive disease repair as EVOR.

CASE SCENARIO:
Endografts for Occlusive Disease (EVOR)

The patient is a 72-year-old woman with severe thigh and buttock claudication at 100 feet ambulation or with prolonged standing. Ankle-brachial indices were 0.7 in the right leg and 0.5 in the left leg. Aortogram demonstrated a single left renal artery, multilevel aortic stenosis and focal bilateral common iliac artery stenosis, figure 17-2. The illustration of the aortoiliac stenosis is seen in figure 17-3. Because of the concomitant aortic and iliac disease, as well as an extensive aortic thrombus, a covered bifurcated endograft was chosen for repair. An Excluder graft size 23 cm x 12 mm x 14 cm was deployed main-body-left via a 16-Fr introducer sheath. Figure 17-4 demonstrates the size relationship of this 16-Fr sheath in a 6 mm

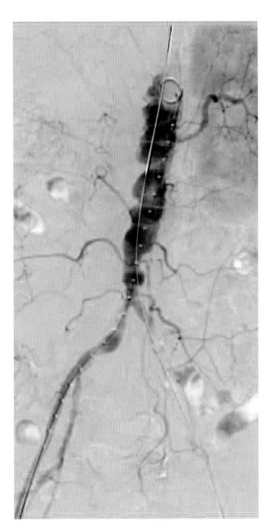

Figure 17-2 Aortogram demonstrating aortoiliac occlusive disease. Visualization of patients left iliac artery is obscured by the sheath.

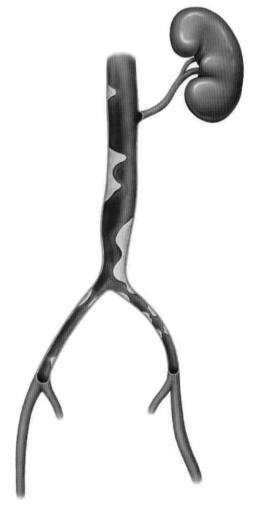

Figure 17-3 Illustration of aortoiliac stenosis and solitary kidney.

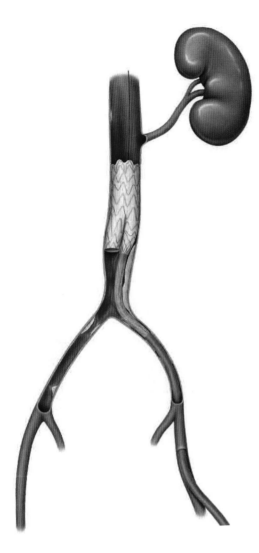

Figure 17-4 Illustration of sheath in aorta with only contralateral gate deployed. The gate should be cannulated prior to deployment of remaining main body graft.

artery with essentially no blood flow around this relatively large sheath. It is important to not remove this sheath from the iliac artery until the contralateral gate has been cannulated and the contralateral graft limb has been placed. If the large right-sided sheath were to cause an iliac dissection/rupture, the contralateral limb fixation will minimize back-bleeding. Additionally, the main body graft is partially deployed so that only the contralateral gate opens but not the ipsilateral

limb. If both the gate and the ipsilateral limb were opened at the same time in a small diameter aorta, the gate could be compressed or "fish-mouthed" against the aortic wall and cannulation of that gate would be difficult, if not impossible. Completion arteriogram after full deployment of the bifurcated endograft demonstrates resolution of aortoiliac stenosis, exclusive of mural thrombus, and no compromise of flow to the solitary renal artery or the internal iliac arteries, as figure 17-5 indicates. Computerized tomographic angiography at one year follow-up is seen in figure 17-6.

CASE DISCUSSION:
Endografts for Occlusive Disease (EVOR)

The last decade has seen exponential growth in the use of endovascular stent grafts to treat aneurysmal disease. Similarly, the scientific literature is replete with studies detailing indications, techniques, and outcomes for endovascular aortic aneurysm repair (EVAR). However, only a relative handful of studies describe the use of endografts for occlusive disease repair (EVOR), and even fewer report the use of bifurcated endografts. The lack of randomized trials and long-term follow-up make it inappropriate to support the widespread use of endografts for occlusive disease. Additionally, the cost of endografts is significantly greater than that of bare-metal stents.

Yet, the theoretical advantages of endografts are intuitive and appealing. Endografts are significantly less invasive than the "open" aortobifemoral bypass and like the aortobifemoral bypass, they can treat long-segment disease. If data from endovascular aortic aneurysm repair (EVAR) were to be extrapolated to endovascular aortic occlusive repair (EVOR), one might expect to see shorter hospital stays and less initial mortality and morbidity as compared with open aortic bypass. Again, this remains unproven. Additionally, complex lesions involving the distal aorta and iliac bifurcation are not well suited for bare-metal stenting and may very well be best treated with bifurcated covered grafts.

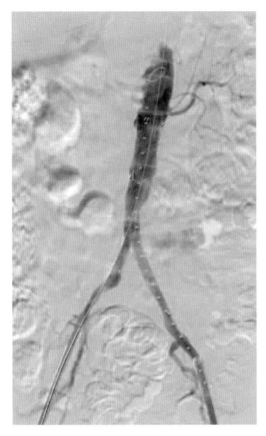

Figure 17-5 Completion aortogram after deployment of bifurcated device. Compare this to the preoperative arteriogram in figure 17-2.

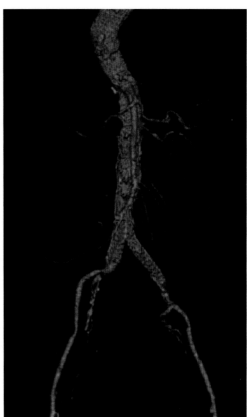

Figure 17-6 Completion computerized tomographic angiogram at one year follow up.

Endovascular aortic occlusive repair (EVOR) may be particularly well-suited for heavily calcified and stenotic aortic lesions. The fabric-covered grafts allow for aggressive angioplasty with less concern for native artery rupture and hemorrhage. Also, EVOR may mitigate against distal embolization (blue toe syndrome) by trapping or excluding mural thrombus against the aortic wall. Theoretically, there may be less risk of prosthetic graft infection than with open aortobifemoral bypass grafting. Whereas endografts are completely intravascular, the aortobifemoral grafts are extravascular and the femoral limbs may easily become infected if the overlying groin incision becomes infected or dehisces.

Finally, in-stent stenosis secondary to myoin-timal hyperplasia with tissue ingrowth through stent interstices is the Achilles' heel of bear-metal stenting. The fabric covered endografts will prevent tissue ingrowth into the lumen of the grafts. This may ultimately prove to be the most significant advantage of endograft repair for occlusive disease.

In summary, the disadvantages of EVOR include: unproven technique with no supporting randomized studies, relatively high cost of the device, and occlusion of arterial side branches. Theoretical advantages of EVOR include: minimally invasive alternative to aortic bypass, the ability to treat long-segment disease, protection against aortic/iliac rupture, reduced distal embolization, low risk of infection, and resistance to intimal hyperplasia.

COMMENTARY

(Scott L. Stevens, Knoxville, TN) Using the same techniques and tools developed for treating aortic aneurysms, this chapter describes an innovative approach for wholly different aortic pathology. Sophisticated imaging, well designed covered stents and elegant catheters, coupled with evolved surgical judgment, have all advanced treatment of aortic occlusive disease. The technique labeled as EVOR allows in-situ aortic bypass though remote femoral access and avoids the physiologic trespass of direct surgical reconstruction.

REFERENCES

1. Domandy JA, Rutherford RB. Management of Peripheral Arterial Disease (PAD) TASC Working Group. Trans Atlantic Inter-Society Consensus (TASC). *J Vasc Surg*. 2000; 31: S1-S296.

2. DeBakey ME, Lawrie GM, Glaeser DH. Patterns of Atherosclerosis and Their Surgical Significance. *Ann Surg*. 1985; 201: 115.

3. Nevelsteen A, Wouters L, Suy R. Long-Term Patency of the Aortofemoral Dacron Graft: A Graft Limb Related Study Over A 25 Year Period. *J Cardiovasc Surg (Torino)*. 1991; 32: 174-180.

4. Szilagyi DE, Elliott JP Jr, Smith RF, et al. A Thirty-Year Survey of the Reconstructive Surgical Treatment of Aortoiliac Occlusive Disease. *J Vasc Surg*. 1986; 3: 421-436.

5. Poulias GE, Polemis L, Skoutas B, et al. Bilateral Aortobifemoral Bypass in the Presence of Aorto-Iliac Occlusive Disease and Factors Determining Results. Experience and Long-Term Follow-Up With 500 Consecutive Cases. *J Cardiovasc Surg*. 1985; 26: 527-538.

6. Dimick JB, Cowan JA Jr, Henke PA, et al. Hospital Volume-Related Differences in Aorto-Bifemoral Bypass Operative Mortality in the United States. *J Vasc Surg*. 2003; 37: 970-975.

7. Reed AB, Conte MS, Donaldson MC, et al. The Impact of Patient Age and Aortic Size on the Results of Aortobifemoral Bypass Grafting. *J Vasc Surg*. 2003; 37: 1219-1225.

8. Sladen JG, Gilmour JL, Wong RW. Cumulative Patency and Actual Palliation in A Patient With Claudication After Aortofemoral Bypass. Prospective Long-Term Follow-Up of 100 Patients. *Am J Surgery*. 1986; 12: 190-195.

9. Mitchell RO, Self SB, Temes GD, and VanDaalen JM. Descending Thoracic Aorta to Femoral Artery Bypass. *J of KY Med Assoc*. 1995; Vol. 93, No.6: 236-239.

10. Yao JST, Pearce WH, eds. *Femorofemoral Bypass: A Twenty-Five Year Experience*. Norwalk, CT: Appleton and Lange Publishers; 1993.

11. Perter BA, Burdick JF, Williams GM. Femoro-Femoral or Ilio-Femoral Bypass for Unilateral Inflow Reconstruction? *Am J Surg*. 1991; 161: 426-430.

12. Harrington ME, Harrington EB, Haimov M, et al. Iliofemoral Versus Femorofemoral Bypass: The Case For An Individualized Approach. *J Vasc Surg*. 1992; 16: 841-854.

13. Rutherford RB, Patt A, Pearce WH. Extra-Anatomic Bypass: A Closer View. *J Vasc Surg*. 1987; 6: 437-446.

14. Christenson JT, Broome A, Norgren L, et al. The Late Results After Axilo-Femoral Bypass in Patients With Leg Ischemia. *J Cardiovas Surg*. 1986; 27: 131-135.

15. Hepp W, DeJunge K, Pallua N. Late Results Following Extraanatomic Bypass Procedure for Chronic Aortoiliac Occlusive Disease. *J Cardiovasc Surg*. 1988; 29: 181-185.

16. Donaldson MC, Louras JC, Bucknam CA. Axillofemoral Bypass: A Tool With A Limited Role. *J Vasc Surg*. 1986; 3: 757-763.

17. Timaran CH, Stevens SL, Freeman MB, Goldman MH. Predictors For Adverse Outcomes After Iliac Angioplasty and Stenting for Limb-Threatening Ischemia. *J Vasc Surg*. 2002; 36: 507-513.

18. Saporal MR, Chatellien G, Long AL, et al. Self-Expandable Stents for the Treatment of Iliac Artery Obstructive Lesions. *AJR Am J Reontgenol*. 1996; 166: 1173-1179.

19. Bosch JL, Hurink MGM. Meta-Analysis of the Results of Percutaneous Transluminal Angioplasty and Stent Placement for Aortoiliac Occlusive Disease. *Radiology*. 1997; 204: 87-96.

20. Henry M, Amor M, Etherenotg, et al. Palmaz Stent in Iliac and Femoropoliteal Arteries: Primary and Secondary Patency in 310 Patients With 2-4 Year Follow-Up. *Radiology*. 1995; 197: 170-174.

21. Powell RJ, Fillinger M, Walsh DB, et al. Predicting Outcomes of Angioplasty and Selective Stenting of Multisegment Iliac Artery Occlusive Disease. *J Vasc Surg*. 2000; 32: 564-56.

22. Powell RJ, Fillinger M, Bettman M, et al. The Durability of Endovascular Treatment of Multisegment Iliac Occlusive Disease. *J Vasc Surg*. 2000; 31: 1178-1184.

23. Group TW. Management of Peripheral Arterial Disease (PAD): TransAtlantic Inter-Society Consensus (TASC). *J Vasc Surg*. 2000; 31 (Suppl): S1-289.

24. Sanchez LA, Marin ML, Veith FJ, et al. Placement of Endovascular Stented Grafts Via Remote Access Sites: A New Approach to the Treatment of Failed Aortoiliofemoral Reconstructions. *Ann Vasc Surg*. 1995; 9: 1-8.

25. Wain RA, Veith FJ, Marin ML, et al. Analysis of Endovascular Graft Treatment for Aortoiliac Occlusive Disease. What Is Its Role Based on Midterm Results? *Ann of Surg*. 1999; 230 (2) 145-151.

26. Lammer J, Dake MD, Bleyn J, et al. Peripheral Arterial Obstruction: Prospective Study of Treatment with a Transluminating Placed Self-Expanding Stent-Graft. International Trial Study Group. *Radiology*. 2000; 217: 95-104.

27. Rzucidlo EM, Powell RJ, Zwolak RM, et al. Early Results of Stent-Grafting to Treat Diffuse Aortoiliac Disease. *J Vasc Surg*. 2003; 37: 1175-80.

28. Ali AJ, Modrall JG, Lopez J, et al. Emerging role of Endovascular Grafts in Complex Aortoiliac Occlusive Disease. *J Vasc Surg*. 2003; 38: 486-491.

29. Karwowski J, Zarins CK. Endografting of the Abdominal Aorta and Iliac Arteries for Occlusive Disease. *J Cardiovas Surg*. 2005; 46: 349-357.

30. Maynar M, Zander T, Qian Z, et al. Bifurcated Endoprosthesis for Treatment of Aortoiliac Occlusive Lesions. *J Endovasc Ther*. 2005; 12: 22-27.

CHAPTER 18

Management of Malignant Superior Vena Cava Syndrome with Covered Endografts

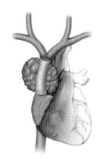

Superior vena cava syndrome is caused by the obstruction of venous blood flow from the upper body to the heart. Symptoms of superior vena cava obstruction may include dyspnea, edema of the arms/head/neck, cyanosis, plethora, and cognitive dysfunction secondary to cerebral edema. Specifically, stenosis or occlusion of the superior vena cava may increase central venous pressure from the normal 2 to 8 mmHg to greater than 40 mmHg.[1-3] The severity of symptoms are related to both the degree of central venous pressure and the rate of onset of the pressure increase.[4]

The etiologies of superior vena cava (SVC) syndrome have been grouped under the general categories of benign or malignant. Benign causes of SVC obstruction have changed over time. In the first 50 years of the 20th century, benign causes of SVC syndrome were almost exclusively thoracic aneurysm, syphilitic aortitis, tuberculosis, granulomatous disease, and mediastinal fibrosis.[1-3,5-6] However, the last 40 years have seen the etiology of benign SVC obstruction change to iatrogenic causes in over 70% of the cases.[3,7-9] Indeed, the majority of cases of benign SVC syndrome are now related to advances in intensive care medicine. In-dwelling central venous catheters for hemodialysis, venous access, and for permanent pacemaker/defibrillators are im-

plicated. It is estimated that five million central venous catheters and 170,000 pacemaker/defibrillators are implanted annually in the United States. Superior vena cava syndrome reportedly occurs in 1% to 3% of patients with long-term central venous catheters and in 0.2% to 3.3% of patients with implanted pacemakers.[3-7, 10-14]

Malignant etiologies are responsive for 65% to 70% of the cases of superior vena cava syndrome.[3] Non-small cell lung cancer is most common and accounts for 50% of the malignant cases of SVC syndrome. Other malignant causes are small cell lung cancer (25%), lymphoma (10%) and metastatic disease (10%).[1, 15-20]

Numerous open surgical techniques have been developed to treat superior vena cava syndrome. Most open techniques require a median sternotomy with subsequent bypass or replacement of the stenotic superior vena cava with a conduit. Various conduits that have been described include polytetrafluoroethylene (PTFE) grafts, spiral vein grafts, superficial femoral vein grafts, and self-constructed pericardial tube grafts.[21-23, 25-27]

SUPERIOR VENA CAVA SYNDROME, CASE 1

The patient is a 35-year-old G2,P0 white female

who is 23 weeks gestation. Core needle biopsy of a bulky mediastinal mass demonstrated non-Hodgkin's lymphoma. The patient developed superior vena cava syndrome with significant edema of the arms, neck and head. She was dyspneic with oxygen saturations of 80% on room air. She had developed perioral cyanosis and was unable to lie recumbent for nearly 48 hours prior to consultation. Chemotherapy and radiation therapy would be detrimental, if not fatal, to her unborn child at 23 weeks gestation. Additionally, the patient refused these options. I recommended an attempt to open the superior vena cava with an endovascular approach and the placement of a covered stent graft.

Figure 18-1 illustrates the mediastinal tumor compressing the superior vena cava. The patient's abdomen was draped with a lead apron and the right femoral vein was percutaneous

cannulated. A 0.035 inch guide wire was slowly advanced through the iliac veins and into the inferior vena cava without the aid of fluoroscopic visualization. The wire was then visualized at the level of the right atrium and with a series of guide catheters the superior vena cava occlusion was traversed and dilated to 8 mm with an angioplasty balloon. A 9 mm diameter x 5 cm length Viabahn endograft was placed across the superior vena cava narrowing and balloon dilated as illustrated in figure 18-2. A covered stent was chosen on the theoretical basis that it would prevent the tumor in-growth that could occur through the intersticies of a bare-metal stent. Additionally, as the superior vena cava was dilated from a luminal diameter of 0 mm to 9 mm, the superior vena cava could be torn or ruptured and a covered graft may protect against catastrophic hemorrhage. However, I am unaware of

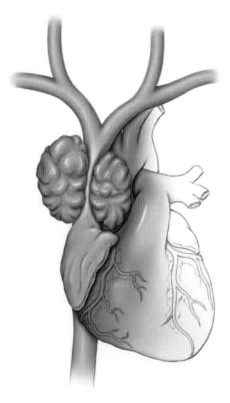

Figure 18-1 Bulky mediastinal tumor compressing superior vena cava.

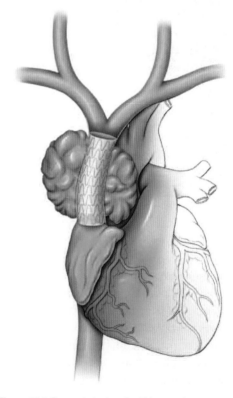

Figure 18-2 Covered stent graft within superior vena cava.

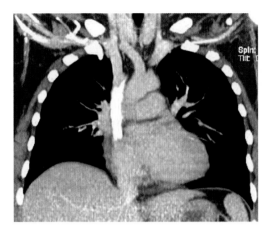

Figure 18-3 CT angiograms demonstrating a patent stent in superior vena cava, coronal view.

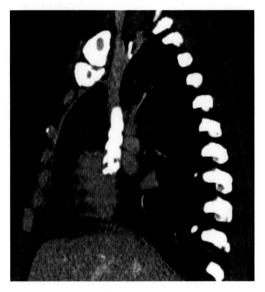

Figure 18-4 CT angiograms demonstrating a patent stent in superior vena cava, sagittal view.

any published reports as to the superiority or even the use of covered grafts in such a situation. The patient's symptoms improved within minutes of stent graft deployment. After successful delivery of her child, the patient proceeded with chemotherapy and radiation therapy and now remains tumor free nearly two and a half years post procedure. Figures 18-3 and 18-4 demonstrate two views of the patent stent graft in the superior vena cava by CT angiogram.

SUPERIOR VENA CAVA SYNDROME, CASE 2

The patient is a 57-year-old white female, non-smoker, with lung cancer and bone metastasis. She had developed progressive dyspnea with head and neck edema over a three week period. Computerized tomography demonstrated no flow lumen within the superior vena cava. I was consulted for consideration of superior vena cava stenting. In the hybrid operating room, multiple attempts were made to cross the superior vena cava obstruction with wires from above via the right axillary vein, and from below via the right femoral vein. Figure 18-5 is a contrast venogram injected from above the obstruction. Figure 18-6 is a venogram with contrast injection from below the superior vena cava obstruction from a catheter in the right atrium. Note that the obstruction is complete. The superior vena cava was eventually opened from below using a series

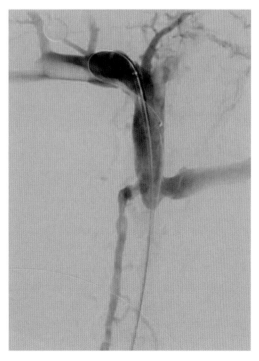

Figure 18-5 Contrast venogram injected from above superior vena cava obstruction. Note enlarged collateral veins in chest.

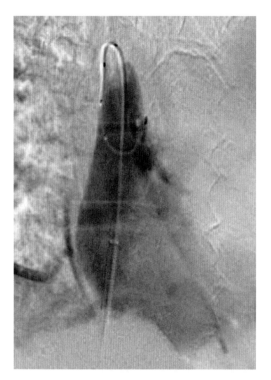

Figure 18-6 Contrast venogram injected into right atrium below superior vena cava obstruction.

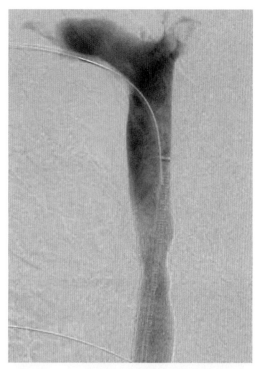

Figure 18-7 Completion vena cavogram demonstrating covered stent and restoration of superior vena cava patency.

of guide catheters through a 90 cm destination sheath. A 13 mm x 5 cm Viabahn covered graft was placed across the obstruction. Figure 18-7 is a completion vena cavogram demonstrating the covered stent restoring caval patency.

CASE DISCUSSIONS:
Superior Vena Cava Syndrome

Endovascular stent placement for superior vena cava syndrome was first described by Charnangavej, et al in 1986.[26] Multiple studies have documented the effectiveness of bare-metal stents at relieving the symptoms of superior vena cava obstruction. The stents most frequently reported for use in the SVC syndrome include the wall stent (Boston Scientific Corp, Natic, MA, U.S.A.), the Gianturco Z stent (Cook, Inc., Bloomington IN, U.S.A.), and the Smart stent (Johnson and Johnson Corp., Warren, NJ, U.S.A.).[29-31]

Stent placement in the stenotic superior vena cava will result in almost immediate increase in right atrial pressure, pulmonary capillary wedge pressure and cardiac output. Although the hemodynamic improvements occur within minutes, the clinical manifestations of superior vena cava syndrome might take 24 to 48 hours for resolution.[32] The rapid efficacy and a low complication rate have allowed superior vena cava stenting to become the first line therapy for benign causes of superior vena cava syndrome.[7]

Superior vena cava syndrome secondary to malignant etiology has traditionally be treated with chemotherapy and radiation therapy. Vena cava stenting had been reserved for failure of chemotherapy or radiation therapy. However, there is now evidence that the paradigm may be shifting in the management of malignant superior vena cava syndrome. Four separate studies with a total of 97 patients have demonstrated 100% effectiveness at relieving the symptoms of superior vena cava obstruction when stenting is used as the initial therapy.[33-36] Superior vena cava stenting is superior to either chemotherapy or radiation therapy in the effectiveness of relieving the vena caval obstructive symptoms. Radiation therapy has been demonstrated to be effective at relieving symptoms in only 63% of patients with non-small cell lung cancer. Improvement in symptoms occurred within three days to two weeks. One-third of patients with non-small cell lung cancer reported no improvement in symptoms after radiation therapy. Additionally, 5% of the non-responders reported a worsening of symptoms after radiation; presumably secondary to pulmonary edema.[15-17, 19, 37-44] Furthermore, autopsy studies have demonstrated a complete or partial superior vena cava patency in only 24% of patients undergoing radiation for symptomatic superior vena cava syndrome.[38]

Chemotherapy alone has been reported to relieve symptoms of superior vena cava obstruction in only 40% of patients with non-small cell lung cancer.[15, 40-41, 45] Two randomized studies and 44 observational studies have concluded that there was no clinical significant difference in the rate of relief of symptoms from superior vena cava obstruction with chemotherapy alone, radiotherapy alone, or combined chemoradiotherapy.[40-41, 43]

Because superior vena cava stenting is extremely effective at relieving symptoms of superior vena cava syndrome, has a rapid response time, and has minimal complications, stenting is becoming a first line therapy for superior vena cava syndrome in many institutions.[32-36, 46-47] I chose a covered graft for superior vena cava stenting on the theoretical basis that it could potentially mitigate against catastrophic hemorrhage and also may impede tumor in-growth, which theoretically may be possible through the intersticies of a bare-metal stent. I am unaware of long-term data or any data regarding the use of a covered stent in this scenario.

COMMENTARY

(Baron L. Hamman, Dallas, TX) The practice of palliative surgery is threatened by the increasing scrutiny of surgical practice. Thoracic surgery is particularly susceptible to this phenomenon because the body of thoracic surgeons in the USA (Society of Thoracic Surgeons – STS found at www.STS.org) have for 25 years built, populated, and edited large patient centric data bases. Data from these data bases are used for improvements in patient care. But because they are now sold to "for profit" public publishing houses for the salacious purpose of "grading" your neighbor, the individual surgeon is now keen to avoid the public scorn of a bad "grade". Palliative surgery suffers.

This case illustrates how treatment of a disastrous complication of an incurable disease can be dramatically improved with the clever off label use of a device. Whether the stent be covered or not covered is unlikely to be of significant importance in the long term outcome of un-resectable or inoperable cancer patients. Arenas in which delay of in growth of tumor or in growth of scar – pannus – is important might affect the decision to use a covered stent. Chronic disease entities such as radiation injury or cicatrix from a foreign body (indwelling line or a pacer wire) would be examples of this circumstance.

Opening the upper body venous system directly to the heart is of great value in the presented case. One may consider using a spiral vein graft technique in a patient who anticipates use of his/her SVC for longer than 7 years.

REFERENCES

1. Chen JC, Bongard F, Klein Sr. A contemporary perspective on superior vena cava syndrome. *Am J Surg.* 1990; 160: 207-211.
2. Parish JM, Marscheke RF Jr, Dines DE, Lee RE. Etiologic considerations in superior vena cava syndrome. *Mayo Clin Proc.* 1981; 56: 407-413.
3. Rice TW, Rodriguez RM, Light RW. The superior vena cava syndrome: Clinical characteristics and evolving etiology. *Medicine (Baltimore).* 2006; 85: 37-42.
4. Wilson D, Detterback FC, Yahalom J. Superior vena cava syndrome with malignant causes. *N Engl J Med.* 2007; 356: 1862-1869.
5. McIntire FT, Sykes EM Jr. Obstruction of the superior vena cava: A review of the literature and report of two personal cases. *Ann Intern Med.* 1949; 30: 925-960.
6. Klassen KP, Andrews NC, Curtis GM. Diagnosis and treatment of superior vena cava obstruction. *AMA Arch Surg.* 1951; 63: 311-325.
7. Rizvi AZ, Kalra M, Bjarnason H, et al. Benign superior vena cava syndrome: Stenting is now the first line of treatment. *J Vasc Surg.* 2008; 47: 372-380.
8. Sheikh MA, Fernandez BB Jr., Gray BH, et al. Endovascular stenting of non-malignant superior vena cava syndrome. *Catheter Cardiov Interv.* 2005; 65: 405-411.
9. Kee ST, Kihoshita L, Razavi MK, et al. Superior vena cava syndrome: Treatment with catheter-directed thrombolysis and endovascular stent placement. *Radiology.* 1998; 206 January (1): 187-193.
10. Gaitini D, Beck-Razi N, Haim N, Brenner B. Prevalence of upper extremity deep venous thrombosis diagnosis by color Doppler duplex sonography in cancer patients with central venous catheters. *J Ultrasound Med.* 2006; 25: 1297-1303.
11. Korkeila P, Nyman K, Ylitalo A, et al. Venous obstruction after pacemaker implantation. *Pacing Clin Eletrophysiol.* 2007; 30: 199-206.
12. Barakat K, Robinson NM, Spurrell RA. Transvenous pacing lead-induced thrombosis: A series of cases with review of the literature. *Cardiology.* 2000; 93: 142-148.
13. Raad I. Intravascular-catheter-related infections. *Lancet.* 1998; 351: 893-898.
14. Rosamond W, Flegal K, Friday G, et al. heart disease and stroke statistics – 2007 update: A report from the American Heart Association Statistics. *Circulation.* 2007; 115: e69-71.
15. Schraufnagel DE, Hill R, Leech JA, Pure JA. Superior vena cava obstruction: Is it a medical emergency? *Am J Med.* 1981; 70: 1169-1174.
16. Nicholson AA, Etles DF, Arnold A, et al. Treatment of malignancy superior vena cava obstruction: Metal stents or radiation therapy. *J Vasc Inter Radio.* 1997; 8: 781-788.
17. Yellin A, Rosen A, Reicheert N, Lieberman Y. Superior vena cava syndrome: The myth-The fact. *Am Rev Respir Dis.* 1990; 141: 1114-1118.
18. Detterback FC, Parsons AM. Thymic Tumors. *Ann Thor Surg.* 2004; 771: 1860-1869.
19. Armstrong BA, Perez CA, Simpson JR, Hedeman MA. Role of irradiation in the management of superior vena cava syndrome. *Int J. Radiat Oncol Biol Phys.* 1987; 13: 531-539.
20. Rice TW, Rodriguez RM, Barnette R, Light RW. Prevalence and characteristics of pleural effusion in superior vena cava syndrome. *Radiology.* 2006; 11: 299-305.
21. Dartevelle PG, Chapelier AR, Pastorin OU, et al. Long-term follow-up after prosthetic replacement of the superior vena cava combined with resection of mediastinal–pulmonary malignant tumors. *J Thorac Cardoivasc Surg.* 1991; 102: 259-265.
22. Magnan PE, Thomas P, Giudicelli R, et al. Surgical reconstruction of the superior vena cava. *Cardiovas Surg.* 1994; 2: 598-604.
23. Gloviczki P, Pairolero PC, Cherry KJ, Hallett JW Jr. Reconstruction of the vena cava and its primary tributaries: A preliminary report. *J Vasc Surg.* 1990; 11: 373-381.
24. Kalra M, Gloviczki P, Andrews JC, et al. Open surgical and endovascular treatment of superior vena cava syndrome caused by non-malignancy disease. *J Vasc Surg.* 2003; 38: 215-223.
25. Doty JR, Flores JH, Doty DB. Superior vena cava obstruction: Bypass using spiral vein graft. *Ann Thorac Surg.* 1999; 67: 1111-1116.
26. Erbella J, Hess PJ, Huber TS. Superior vena cava bypass with superficial femoral vein for benign superior vena cava syndrome. *Ann Vasc Surg.* 2006; 20: 834-838.
27. Reardon MJ and Davies MG. Central venous stenosis – Endovascular and surgical treatments. *Methodist DeBakey Cardiovasc J.* 2009; vol (5) 4: 32-35.
28. Charnsongaves C, Carrasco CH, Wallace S, et al. Stenosis of the vena cava: Preliminary assessment of treatment with expandable metal stents. *Radiology.* 1986; 161: 295-298.
29. Urruticoechea A, Mesia R, Dominguey J, et al. Treatment of malignant superior vena cava syndrome by endovascular stent insertion: Experience on 52 patients with lung cancer. *Lung Cancer.* 2004; 43: 209-214.
30. Courtheoux P, Alkofen B, Refai M, et al. Stent placement in superior vena cava syndrome. *Ann Thorac Surg.* 2003; 75: 158-161.
31. Ganeshan A, Quen Hon L, Warakaulle D, et al. Superior vena cava stenting for SVC obstruction: Current status. *E J. Radiol.* 2009; 71: 343-349.
32. Yamagami T, Nakamura T, Kato T, et al. Hemodynamic changes after self expandable metallic stent therapy for superior vena cava syndrome. *Am J Roentgenol.* 2002; 178: 635-639.
33. Lopez-Muiz JIC, Garcia GL, Lanciego C, et al. Treatment of superior and inferior vena cava syndrome of malignant cause with Wallstent catheter placed percutaneous. *Am J Clin Oncol.* 1997; 20: 293-297.
34. Lanciego C, Chaucon JL, Julia A, et al. Stenting as first option for endovascular treatment of malignant superior vena cava syndrome. *Am J Roentgenol.* 2001; 177: 585-593.

35. Gross CM, Kramer J, Waigand J, et al. Stent implantation in patients with superior vena cava syndrome. *Am J Roentgenol.* 1997; 169: 429-432.

36. Chatziioannou A, Alexopoulos T, Mourikis D, et al. Stent therapy for malignant superior vena cava syndrome: Should be first line therapy or simple adjuct to radiotherapy. *Eur J Radoi.* 2003; 47: 247-250.

37. Ostler P J, Clarke DP, Watkinson AF, Gaze MN. Superior vena cava obstruction: A moderate management strategy. *Clin oncol.* 1997; 9: 83-89l

38. Ahmann FR. A reassessment of the clinical implications of the superior vena cava syndrome. *J Clin Oncol.* 1984; 2: 961-969.

39. Chan RH, Daw AR, Yu E, et al. Superior vena cava obstruction in small-cell lung cancer. *Int J Radiat Oncol Biol Phys.* 1997; 38: 513-5290.

40. Rowell NP, Gleeson FV. Steroids, radiotherapy, chemotherapy and stents for superior vena caval obstruction in carcinoma of the bronchus: A systematic review. *Clin Oncol.* 2002; 14: 338-351.

41. Spiro SG, Shah S, Harper PG, et al. Treatment of obstruction of the superior vena cava by combination chemotherapy with and without irradiation in small-cell carcinoma of the bronchus. *Thorax.* 1983; 38: 501-505.

42. Anderson PR, Coia LR. Fractionation and outcomes with palliative radiation therapy. *Semin Radiat Oncol.* 2000; 10: 191-199.

43. Pereira JR, Martins SJ, Ikari FK, et al. Neoadjuvant chemotherapy vital signs radiotherapy alone for superior vena cava syndrome (SVCS) due to non-small cell lung cancer (NSCL): Preliminary results of randomized Phage II trial. *Eur J Cancer.* 1999; 35: suppl 4: 260.

44. Wurschmidt F, Bunemann H, Heilmann HP. Small cell lung cancer with and without superior vena cava syndrome: A multivariate analysis or prognostic factors in 408 cases. *Int J Radiat Oncol Biol Phys.* 1995; 33: 77-82.

45. Sculier JP, Evans WK, Feld R, et al. Superior vena cava obstruction syndrome in small cell lung cancer. *Cancer.* 1986; 57: 847-851.

46. Nagata T, Makutani S, Uchida H, et al. Follow-up results of 71 patients undergoing metallic stent placement for the treatment of a malignant obstruction of the superior vena cava. *Cardiovasc Int Radiol.* 2007; 30: 959-967.

47. Bierdruger E, Lampman T, Kato T, et al. Endovascular stenting in neoplastic superior vena cava syndrome prior to chemotherapy or radiotherapy. *Neth J Med.* 2005; 63: 20-23.

CHAPTER 19

Endovascular Repair of an Isolated Common Iliac Artery Aneurysm with a Bifurcated Endograft

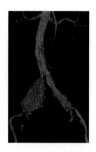

Common iliac artery aneurysms (CIAA) are usually associated with an abdominal aortic aneurysm. Isolated common iliac aneurysms are actually not common. One study concluded that the incidence of isolated CIAAs was 1 in 6,000 autopsy population.[1] They are generally found in older men and the etiology is believed to be similar to that of abdominal aortic aneurysms. Older literature indicated pain as the primary symptom leading to diagnosis; however, more recent studies conclude that most CIAAs are asymptomatic when diagnosed.[2, 3] A common iliac artery is defined as aneurysmal at a diameter greater 1.8 cm.[4]

Just as in the case of abdominal aortic aneurysms, CIAAs have a natural history of progressive enlargement and rupture. They are estimated to enlarge at a rate of 0.5 to 1.1 mm per year with an increased rate of growth as their diameter increases.[5] At a diameter of 5 cm, the risk of rupture is 75% per year. Isolated CIAAs should be repaired at a diameter of 3 to 3.5 cm or at 2.5 cm if present at the time of concomitant aortic aneurysm repair.[5, 6] In a study of 473 CIAAs by Sandhu and Pipinos, the operative mortality for emergency surgery or rupture was 28% and for elective surgery was 5%.[7]

CASE SCENARIO:
Common Iliac Artery Aneurysms

The patient is a 60-year-old man with an incidental finding of a 4.8 cm right common iliac artery aneurysm identified during a cardiac catheterization. The computerized tomographic angiogram seen in figures 19-1 and 2 demonstrate the right CIAA very close to the aortic bifurcation. Options of open versus endovascular repair were discussed with the patient and he strongly

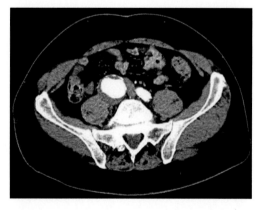

Figure 19-1 Axial CT scan of the right common iliac artery aneurysm.

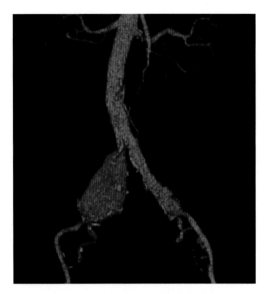

Figure 19-2 Three dimension CT-angiogram of right common iliac artery aneurysm.

preferred an endovascular approach. Because of the proximity of the aneurysm to the aortic bifurcation, a straight covered endograft would be inappropriate as there was an inadequate length of "normal" iliac artery to provide a proximal landing zone. A bifurcated endograft would provide 3-points of seal zone and should be effective.

An intraoperative arteriogram via the right femoral artery demonstrates the aneurysm, figure 19-3. Three embolic coils were placed into the right internal iliac artery to prevent a type-II endoleak. A bifurcated graft was placed via the right femoral artery with the necessary extension limbs. Completion aortogram demonstrates the deployed bifurcated graft and the complete exclusion of the iliac aneurysm, figure 19-4.

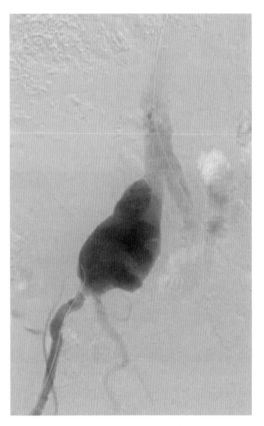

Figure 19-3 Intraoperative arteriogram of the iliac aneurysm.

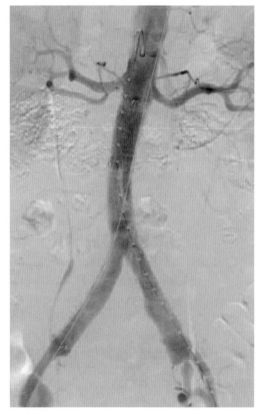

Figure 19-4 Intraoperative Aortogram after placement of bifurcated endograft with exclusion of aneurysm.

CASE DISCUSSION:
Common Iliac Artery Aneurysms

Although much less common than aortic aneurysms, ruptured iliac artery aneurysms are nearly as lethal. Advances in endovascular therapy have allowed for the repair of iliac aneurysms with minimal operative risk. However, the long-term durability of endovascular repairs in this situation is not yet known. There is a paucity of long-term data regarding the use of a bifurcated endograft to treat proximal CIAAs. Clearly the added expense of a bifurcated device should be considered. The patient remains under surveillance, but in this scenario I propose that problems such as graft migration and endoleak would be much less with the use a bifurcated graft for an abdominal aortic aneurysm.

REFERENCES

1. Brunkwall J, Hauksson H, Bengtsson H, et al. Solitary Aneurysms of the Iliac Arterial Systems: An Estimate of Their Frequency of Occurrence. *Journal of Vascular Surgery.* October 1989; 10 (4): 381-384.

2. Krupski WC, Selzman CH, Floridia R, et al. Contemporary Management of Isolated Iliac Aneurysms. *Journal of Vascular Surgery.* July 1998; 28 (1): 1-11; Discussion 11-13.

3. Richardson JW, Greenfield LJ. Natural History and Management of Iliac Aneurysms. *Journal of Vascular Surgery.* August 1988; 8 (2): 165-171.

4. Johnston KW, Rutherford RB, Tilson MD, et al. Suggested Standards for Reporting on Arterial Aneurysms. Society for Vascular Surgery and North American Chapter International Society for Cardiovascular Surgery. *Journal of Vascular Surgery.* March 1999; 13 (3): 452-458.

5. Santilli SM, Wernsing SE, Lee ES. Expansion Rates and Outcomes for Iliac Artery Aneurysms. *Journal of Vascular Surgery.* January 2000; 31 (1 pt 1): 114-121.

6. Lowry SF, Kraft RO. Isolated Aneurysms of the Iliac Artery. *Archives of Surgery.* November 1978; 113 (11): 1289-1293.

7. Cronenwett JL, Johnston KW, eds. *In Rutherford's Vascular Surgery.* 7th ed. Chapter 128. Philadelphia, PA: Sanders Elsevier; 2010.

CHAPTER 20

Endovascular Repair of a Ruptured 8 cm Internal Iliac Artery Aneurysm, 16 Years after the Open Repair of a Ruptured Abdominal Aortic Aneurysm

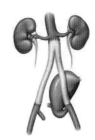

Isolated internal iliac artery aneurysms are relatively rare and may represent less than 1% of intra-abdominal aneurysms. Approximately 80% of patients with internal or common iliac artery aneurysms also have an abdominal aortic aneurysm.[1-4] Common iliac artery aneurysms are defined as aneurysmal when their diameter reaches 1.8 cm. Internal iliac arteries are aneurysmal, by definition, at a diameter of 0.8 cm.[5] Most iliac aneurysms are found in older males and are believed to have a degenerative etiology similar to abdominal aortic aneurysms.[2, 6]

The natural history of iliac aneurysms is not as well defined as that of abdominal aortic aneurysms. However, they clearly progress through expansion and rupture over time. It is known that the annual risk of rupture of a 5 cm common iliac artery aneurysm is 75%.[7, 8] Ruptured common iliac artery aneurysms have an operative mortality rate of 40%.[7, 9] It is recommended that common iliac artery aneurysms be repaired at a diameter of 2.5 cm when there is concomitant repair of an infrarenal abdominal aortic aneurysm.[7, 10, 11] Repair of isolated common iliac artery aneurysms should be at a diameter of 3.0-3.5 cm.[7] Much less is known about isolated internal iliac artery aneurysms, but they present with rupture 40% of the time and have a known operative mortality rate of 31%.[7, 10, 12]

CASE SCENARIO:
Ruptured Internal Iliac Artery Aneurysm

A 79-year-old white man presented to the emergency department with a six-hour history of severe left hip and back pain. Sixteen years prior, the patient has undergone repair of a ruptured infrarenal abdominal aortic aneurysm using a bifurcated Dacron graft from the aorta to the origin of the external iliac arteries bilaterally. The common iliac arteries had been over-sewn proximally and thus blood flow to the pelvis was preserved via the internal iliac arteries.

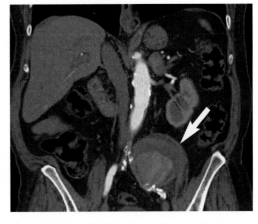

Figure 20-1 Coronal CT angiogram demonstrating 8 cm left-internal iliac artery aneurysm, white arrow.

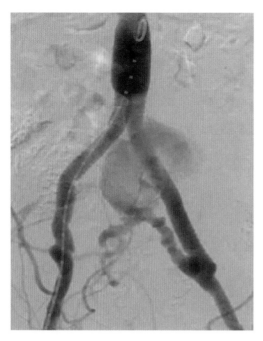

Figure 20-2 Intraoperative arteriogram of ruptured left internal iliac artery aneurysm.

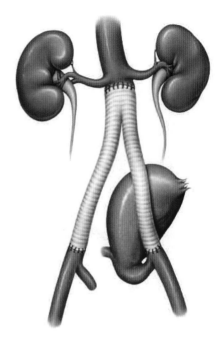

Figure 20-3 Illustration of ruptured left internal iliac artery aneurysm.

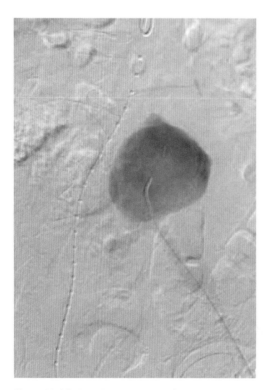

Figure 20-4 Catheter in aneurysm sac for coil embolization.

Computerized tomographic angiography demonstrated an 8.3 cm fluid collection around the left internal iliac artery with a density consistent with blood, figure 20-1. It was unclear as to whether this represented a true internal iliac artery rupture, or a ruptured pseudoaneurysm at the previous graft anastomosis. Because of the patient's advanced age and reoperative status, an endovascular approach was planned.

Intraoperative arteriogram confirmed a true internal iliac artery rupture, figure 20-2. Figure 20-3 illustrates the anatomy of the rupture in relation to the previous graft. Figure 20-4 shows a catheter within the aneurysm sac for the delivery of embolizing coils. A Viabahn covered stent graft, size 11 mm x 10 cm length, was placed from the distal end of the previous Dacron graft, spanning the anastomosis, and landing in the native external iliac artery. This isolates and excludes the internal iliac artery aneurysm from antegrade blood flow. Figure 20-5 is the completion intraoperative arteriogram demonstrating occlusion of the aneurysm sac and no extravasation of contrast. Figure 20-6 is

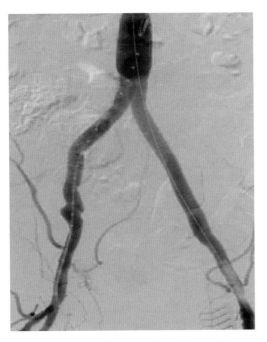

Figure 20-5 Completion intraoperative arteriogram after stent graft deployment, contrast no longer visible in aneurysm sac.

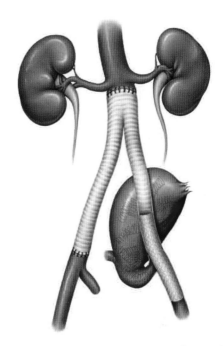

Figure 20-6 Illustration of completed repair of ruptured internal iliac artery aneurysm.

the artists illustration of the completed procedure. Figure 20-7 is a CT angiogram 13 months post procedure demonstrating the stability of this repair.

DISCUSSION:
Ruptured Internal Iliac Artery Aneurysm

Most series report an operative mortality of 30% for ruptured internal iliac artery aneurysms and greater than 50% for ruptured abdominal aortic aneurysms.[7, 10, 12] Certainly, in a patient with advanced age and a hostile abdomen from previous repair of a ruptured infrarenal aortic aneurysm, the operative mortality might be expected to be even higher. This patient is fortunate to have survived two aneurysm ruptures. In this case scenario, an endovascular approach was used and would appear to be favored over open surgery. Two studies have attempted to compare the outcomes of open versus endovascular therapy for internal iliac aneurysms.[3, 13] Both studies had small numbers of patients, and at this time definitive recommendations are lacking as to which is the procedure of choice.

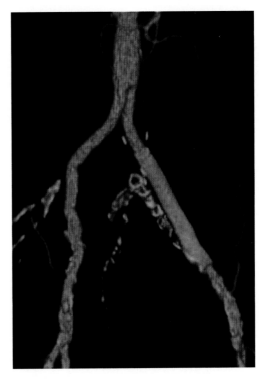

Figure 20-7 CT angiogram 13 months post repair of ruptured internal iliac artery aneurysm.

REFERENCES

1. Boules TN, Selzer, Stanziale SF, et al. Endovascular Management of Isolated Iliac Artery Aneurysms. *J Vasc Surg.* 2006; 44: 29-37.

2. Richardson JW, Greenfield LJ: Natural History and Management of Iliac Aneurysms. *J Vasc Surg.* 1988; 8: 165-171.

3. Pitoulias GA, Donas KP, Schulte S, et al. Isolated Iliac Artery Aneurysms: Endovascular Versus Open Elective Repair. *J Vasc Surg.* 2007; 46: 648-654.

4. Armon WP, Wenham PW, Whitaker SC, et al. Common Iliac Artery Aneurysms in Patients With Abdominal Aortic Aneurysms. *Eur J Vasc Endovasc Surg.* 1998; 15: 255-257.

5. Johnston KW, Rutherford RB, Tilson MD, et al. Suggested Standards for Reporting on Arterial Aneurysms. Subcommittee on Reporting Standards for Arterial Aneurysms. Society for Vascular Surgery and North American Chapter, International Society for Cardiovascular Surgery. *J Vasc Surg.* March 1991; 13 (3); 452-458.

6. Breakwall J, Hauksson H, Bengtsson H, et al. Solitary Aneurysm of the Iliac Arterial System: An Estimate of Their Frequency of Occurrence. *J Vasc Surg.* Oct 1989; 10 (4): 381-384.

7. Santilli SM, Wernsing SE, Lee ES. Expansion Rates and Outcomes for Iliac Artery Aneurysms. *J Vasc Surg.* Jan 2000: 31 (1pt1): 114-131.

8. Kalkoi Y, Basaran M, Aydin U, et al. The Surgical Treatment of Arterial Aneurysms in Behcet Disease: A Report of 16 Patients. *J Vasc Surg.* Oct 2005: 42 (4): 673-677.

9. Krupski WC, Selzman CH, Floridia R, et al. Contemporary Management of Isolated Iliac Aneurysms. *J Vasc Surg.* Jul 1998; 28 (1): 1-11 discussion 11-13.

10. Sala F, Hassen-Khodja R, Branchereau P, et al. Outcome of Common Iliac Arteries After Aortoiliac Graft Placement During Elective Repair of Infrarenal Abdominal Aortic aneurysms. *J Vasc Surg.* Nov 2002; 36 (5) 982-987.

11. Hassen-Khodja R, Feugier P, Favre JP, et al. Outcome of Common Iliac Arteries After Straight Aortic Tube-Graft Placement During Elective Repair of Infrarenal Abdominal Aortic Aneurysms. *J Vasc Surg.* Nov 2006; 44 (5): 943-948.

12. Dix FP, Titi M, Al-Khaffar H. The Isolated Iliac Artery Aneurysm – A Review. *Eur J Vascular Endovasc Surg.* Aug 2005; 30 (2) 119-129.

13. Chaer RA, Barbato JE, Lin SCm et al. Isolated Iliac Artery Aneurysms: A Contemporary Comparison of Endovascular and Open Repair. *J Vasc Surg.* 2008; 47: 708-713.

CHAPTER 21

Hybrid Endograft Repair of an Aberrant Right Subclavian Artery in a Patient with Dysphagia Lusoria

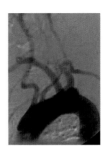

An aberrant origin of the right subclavian artery is one of the most common congenital anomalies of the aortic arch and occurs in 0.5% to 2% of the population.[1-4] The aberrant right subclavian artery (ARSA) originates in the left chest as the most distal branch of the thoracic aorta and courses posterior to the esophagus en route to the right arm, figure 21-1. A saccular outpunching at the base of

the ARSA is known as the Diverticulum of Kommerell. This diverticulum is a remnant of the primitive right dorsal aorta and is present in 60% of patients with an ARSA.[5, 6]

A small percentage of patients with an ARSA will have dysphagia secondary to posterior compression of the esophagus. The incidence of dysphagia associated with an ARSA is unknown but in

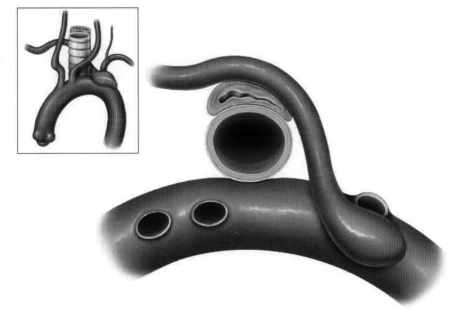

Figure 21-1 Aberrant right subclavian artery originating from aortic arch distal to left subclavian artery. Note course of artery posterior to esophagus and compressing esophagus.

most patients symptoms do not occur until after 40 years of age. The term dysphagia lusoria (freak of nature) was first used by Bayden in 1792 to describe dysphagia caused by the ARSA compressing the esophagus.

True aneurysms of ARSAs are rare with 32 patients described in a review of the literature by Austin and Wolfe. They reported a perioperative mortality of 25%.[9] The largest single center study of symptomatic or aneurysmal ARSAs reported a 26.9% operative mortality rate.[10, 11] The mortality of a ruptured ARSA is reported at 100%.[12]

Esophageal manometric studies in symptomatic patients are nearly always abnormal. However, a specific and reproducible component of the manometry that can be diagnostic of an ARSA has not been identified.[8]

The diagnosis of dysphagia lusoria can be made by barium contrast esophagram, which demonstrates a characteristic posterior indention of the esophagus at approximately the level of the 4th thoracic vertebra. Also, CT angiography will show that ARSA coursing posterior to the compressed esophagus. The below case scenario will describe the diagnosis and subsequent hybrid endovascular management of a patient with dysphagia lusoria.

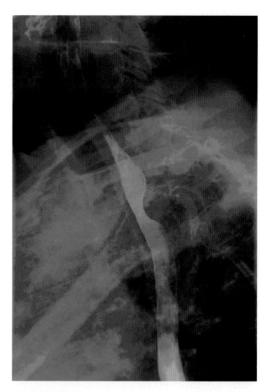

Figure 21-2 Barium contrast esophagram with posterior indentation from ARSA.

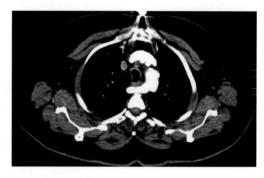

Figure 21-3 Axial CT angiogram images demonstrating esophageal compression by ARSA.

CASE SCENARIO:
Dysphagia Lusoria

The patient is a 60-year-old woman with a 3-year history of dysphagia. She also has significant pulmonary insufficiency having begun smoking at 4 years of age with an increase to 20 cigarettes per day by 10 years of age. Prior to referral for surgical therapy, she had been evaluated by a gastroenterologist and an otolaryngologist. Esophageal manometry was abnormal with frequent retrograde peristaltic waves and overall ineffective motility while maintaining a normal lower esophageal sphincter pressure. A barium contrast esophagram demonstrated a posterior indentation of the esophagus at the level of the 4th thoracic vertebra, figure 21-2. A computerized tomographic angiogram demonstrated an ARSA coursing pos-

terior to the compressed esophagus, figure 21-3.

A thoracic aortagram was done prior to the day of surgery to aid in case planning. I had concerns that the CTA alone would be inadequate to fully evaluate the vertebral arteries. Indeed the left vertebral artery was large and dominate, and arose deep in the chest on the proximal left subclavian artery (LSCA). The right vertebral artery was

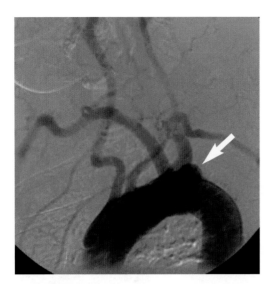

Figure 21-4 Thoracic aortagram with ARSA. Note double-density bulbous enlargement at base of ARSA (arrow).

diminutive but was relatively lateral and it would potentially be easy to ligate the ARSA proximal to both the right carotid to subclavian bypass and the origin of the right vertebral artery. Additionally, the thoracic aortagram demonstrated the origins of the left subclavian artery and the ARSA were in extremely close proximity, and it would be necessary to cover both of these arteries with the thoracic endograft. The thoracic aortagram is seen in figure 21-4. Note also the double-density which is the enlarged bulbous base of the ARSA. The illustration of this aortagram is figure 21-5.

Under general anesthesia with electro-encephalographic (EEG) monitoring, bilateral carotid artery to subclavian artery bypasses were constructed with ring-supported PTFE Propaten grafts. No deleterious EEG changes were encountered with carotid clamping. The ARSA was ligated proximal to the origin of the right vertebral artery. The right femoral artery was exposed by cutdown and a 22-Fr sheath was introduced into the abdominal aorta over a super stiff guidewire. A C-TAG thoracic endograft size 31 mm by 10 cm was deployed in the thoracic aorta just distal to the left carotid artery and covering the origins of the LSCA and the ARSA. An intraoperative aortagram

demonstrated some "late" contrast filling the ARSA. I postulated that there was an area of shared-ostium between the LSCA and ARSA. Embolic coils were introduced by directly cannulating the distal ARSA just proximal to the ligated right vertebral artery. Unfortunately, the small right vertebral artery was then ligated in order to control bleeding that resulted from the coiling maneuver. No abnormal EEG changes were encountered. The coiling proved effective and the completed procedure with bilateral carotid to subclavian bypasses and a C-TAG endograft occluding the origins of both subclavian arteries is illustrated in figure 21-6. The intraoperative arteriogram demonstrates no contrast agent in the ARSA, figure 21-7. The CTA prior to patient discharge confirms the poster operative arteriographic findings with absence of blood flow in the ARSA, figure 21-8.

CASE DISCUSSION:
Dysphagia Lusoria

The first successful surgical repair of dysphagia lusoria was reported by Gross in 1946.[16] Since then a variety of open surgical approaches have been reported and include thoracotomy, median sternotomy, cervical incisions, and even the use of cardiopulmonary bypass. Recently, there have been reports describing hybrid procedures which combine extra-anatomic arterial bypass with endovascular aortic stent grafts.[11, 13-15] Hybrid procedures have the potential advantage of being less invasive and have a lower operative mortality in the very few cases reported.

For the specific patient presented in the above case scenario, a minimally invasive alternative was appealing as the patient had significant pulmonary insufficiency. It might be argued that the ARSA could simply be ligated proximal and distal to the esophagus via a cervical incision and the dysphagia symptoms would resolve and a thoracic endograft would be unnecessary. However, such an approach in this patient would leave the enlarged stump at the base of the ligated ARSA that could degenerate into an aneurysm. Intravascular occluding devices

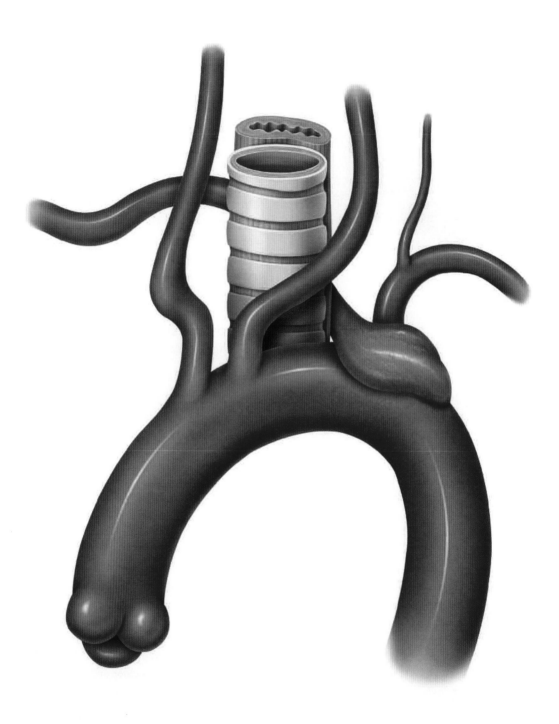

Figure 21-5 Illustration of the aortagram seen in figure 21-4. Note retroesophageal course of aberrant right subclavian artery and its bulbous origin as a Diverticulum of Kommerell.

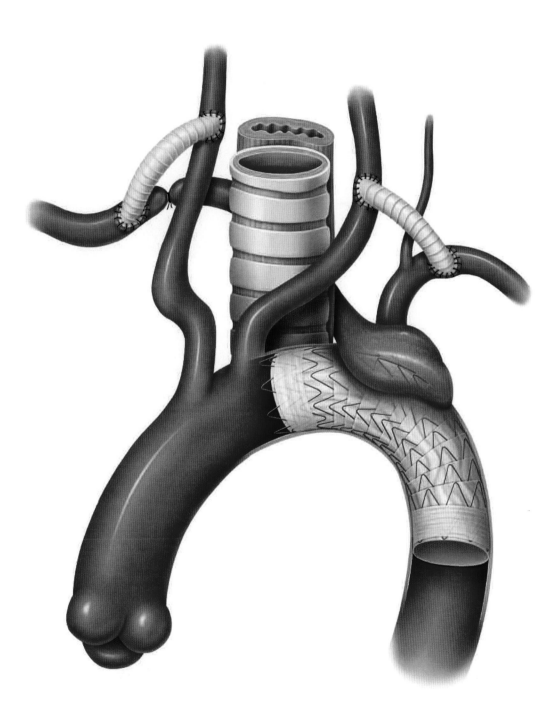

Figure 21-6 Illustration of postoperative arteriogram seen in figure 21-7. Right and left carotid artery to subclavian artery bypass and endoaortic exclusion of the origins of the ARSA and LSCA.

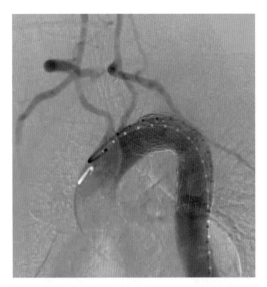

Figure 21-7 Intraoperative aortagram after bilateral carotid to subclavian bypass, ligation of distal ARSA, and deployment of C-TAG in aorta. Note near complete obliteration of ARSA.

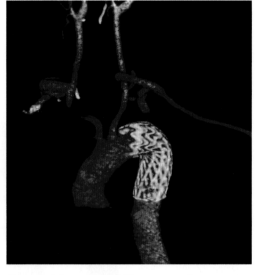

Figure 21-8 Post operative CT angiogram after bilateral carotid to subclavian bypass, ligation of distal ARSA, and deployment of C-TAG. The ARSA is void of contrast and no longer visible.

have been placed in the proximal ARSA as a method of ligating the artery internally at the origin from the aorta; however, sealing the aorta from within by endografting is conceptually more appealing. The thoracic endograft leaves virtually no chance of the Kommerell Diverticu-lum becoming pressurized. Although long-term follow-up date are lacking, endovascular occlusion of a symptomatic ARSA, with or without aneurysm, by means of a thoracic endograft combined with distal ligation is an alternative to open repair.[17]

REFERENCES

1. Turkenburg JL, Versteegh MI, Shaw PK. Case Report: Aneurysm of an aberrant right subclavian artery diagnosed with MR imaging. *Clin Radiol.* 1994; 49: 837-839.

2. Kadir S. *Regional anatomy of the thoracic aorta.* In: Kadir S. Atlas of normal and variant angiographic anatomy. Philadelphia, PA: WB Saunders; 1991.

3. Boening A, Dresler C, Haverich A, et al. Two-stage repair of a combined aneurysm of the descending aorta and the aberrant right subclavian artery. *Eur J Cardiothorac Surg.* 1999; 16: 246-248.

4. Freed K, Low VHS. The aberrant subclavian artery. *AJR Am J Roentgenol.* 1997; 168: 481-484.

5. Davidian M, Kee ST, Kato N, et al. Aneurysm of an aberrant right subclavian artery: Treatment with PTFE covered stent graft. *J Vasc Surg.* 1998; 28: 335-339.

6. Van Son AAM, Konstantin OVI, Burckhard F. Kommerell and Kommerell's diverticulum. *Tex Heart Inst J.* 2002; 29: 109-112.

7. Bayford. An account of singular and of obstructed deglutition. *Memories Med Soc of London.* 1794; 2: 275-286.

8. Janssen M, Baggen MGA, Veen HF, et al. Dysphagia Lusoria: Clinical aspects, manometric findings, diagnosis, and therapy. *Amer J of Gastroenterology.* 2000; 95 (6): 1411-1416.

9. Austin EH, Wolfe WG. Aneurysm of aberrant subclavian artery with a review of the literature. *J Vasc Surg.* 1985; 2: 571-577.

10. Keiffer E, Bahnini A, Kaskas F. Aberrant subclavian artery: Surgical Treatment in thirty-three adult patients. *J Vasc Surg.* 1994; 19:100-109.

11. Tosenovsky P, Quigley F, Golledge J. Hybrid repair of an aberrant right subclavian artery with Kommerells Diverticulum. *Eur Soc Vasc Surg.* 2010; 19 e31-e33.

12. Kopp R, Wizgall I, Kreuzer E, et al. Surgical and endovascular treatment of symptomatic with right subclavian artery (arteria lusoria). *Vascular.* 2007; 15 (2): 84-91.

13. Shennib H, Dietrich EB, Novel approaches for the treatment of the aberrant right subclavian artery and its aneurysm. *J Vasc Surg.* 2008 May; 47 (5): 1066-1070.

14. Attman T, Brandt M, Muller-Hulsbeck S, et al. Two-stage surgical and endovascular treatment of an aberrant right subclavian (lusoria) artery. *Eur J Cardiothorac Surg.* 2005; 27: 1125-1127.

15. Lacroix V, Astarci P, Pilippe D, et al. Endovascular treatment of an aneurysmal aberrant right subclavian artery. *J Endovasc Ther.* 2003 Apr 10; 10 (2): 190-194.

16. Gross RE. Surgical treatment of dysphagia lusoria. *Ann Surg.* 1946; 124: 532-534.

17. Cronenwett JL, Johnston KW, eds. *Rutherford's vascular surgery.* 7th ed. Vol 2, Chap 137, P 2134. Philadelphia, PA: Saunders Elsevier; 2010.

CHAPTER 22

Left Ventricle Apicoaortic Valved Conduit

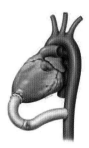

AORTIC VALVULAR STENOSIS

Aortic valve stenosis is the most commonly acquired degenerative valve disease and the incidence of aortic valve stenosis increases with increasing patient age. Currently, the elderly represent the largest segment in the United States population. Therefore, it is deductive that the overall incidence of aortic valve stenosis is increasing.[1] For patients with symptomatic aortic valve stenosis aortic valve replacement has long been shown to prolong life, even among octogenarians.[2-7] However, some studies have indicated that as many as 60% of octogenarians with symptomatic aortic stenosis are not referred to a surgeon either because of a real or perceived belief that they are at a prohibitive surgical risk.[4, 8-11] Indeed traditional aortic valve replacement surgery carries a substantial risk in the elderly. The risk is especially significant in a particular subset of the population. Patients with extensively calcified (porcelain) aorta are at prohibitive risk for aortic cross-clamping and wound require a period of hypothermic circulatory arrest for traditional valve replacement. Additionally, patients who have had prior coronary bypass surgery are at increased risk because of potential injury to the proximal bypass grafts attached to the aorta. Other studies have indicated a 12% incidence of renal failure among elderly patients undergoing conventional aortic valve replacement.[6] Recent developments with transfemoral aortic (TAVI) valves are promising; however, these valves are not widely available, are associated with an increased risk of stroke, and have access issues in patients with peripheral vascular disease.

CASE SCENARIO:
Apicoaortic Valved Conduit

The patient is an 84-year-old woman with multiple hospital admissions for acute on chronic systolic and diastolic congestive heart failure. Echocardiogram indicated critical aortic valve stenosis with a valve area of 0.5 cm^2 and a peak valve gradient of 80 mmHg. The patient had concomitant 3-4+ mitral valvular insufficiency. Although a lifelong non-smoker, the patient had been on home oxygen for greater than one year and had a preoperative PaO2 of 51mmHg on 4 liters per minute of supplemental oxygen. Left heart catheterization demonstrated no significant coronary artery disease.

The patient had a general decompensation in her overall health during the previous six months and was significantly frail. The patient was a prohibitive operative risk for traditional aortic valve replacement and mitral valve repair. Multiple options were discussed including transfer of the patient to a facility for a research with the TAVI valve consideration. The patient agreed to aortic valve bypass by using an apical to aortic valved conduit.

In the operating room, a double-lumen endotracheal tube was placed. A Swan-Ganz catheter demonstrated a pulmonary artery pressure of 68-70 mmHg while the systemic systolic blood pressure was 118 mmHg. With the patient in the left thoracotomy position, a small incision was made between the fifth and sixth intercostal space to digitally palpate for the apex of the heart. This helps to determine the appropriate interspace for best exposure to the cardiac apex. A 16 mm valved-conduit was sutured to a 14 mm apical connector (Medtronic Inc., Santa Rosa, CA) on the back table. Ten-thousand units of heparin were administered intravenously and a partial occluding clamp was placed on the descending thoracic aorta. The 16 mm conduit was anastomosed to the aorta with 4-0 monofilament suture. The clamp was removed to back-fill and de-air the conduit. Braided 2-0 sutures with pledgets were placed in quadrants through the myocardium of the left ventricular apex using a technique described by Brown and Gammie.[20] A circular knife was used to core the myocardium in the center of the quadrant created by the pledgeted sutures. Immediately upon placing the connector in the myocardium, the left ventricular pressure is relieved as there is a double-outlet via the native aortic valve and the new conduit valve. The reduced left ventricular pressure also improves the mitral valvular regurgitation by at least one grade. To reduce bleeding complications and to prevent undue ventricular damage, the connector should not be oversized. The new post-procedure valve area is not just that of a new valve in the conduit, but also the added valve area of the residual native valve. Further stenosis of the native valve does not occur.[12]

This 84-year-old patient on 4 liters of oxygen preoperatively was extubated post procedure while still in the operating room and remained extubated throughout her hospital stay. Figure 22-1 illustrates the completed conduit procedure and figure 22-2 is a CT angiogram obtained prior to patient discharge.

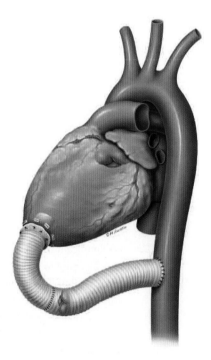

Figure 22-1 Illustration of valved conduit between the left ventricular apex and descending thoracic aorta.

CASE DISCUSSION:
Apicoaortic Valved Conduit

The creation of an apical to aortic conduit was first performed successfully in 1962.[13] This procedure was generally abandoned due to the high degree of difficulty and the emergence of conventional valve replacement surgery which was not as technically demanding. Yet, the creation of a double-outlet left ventricle to relieve outflow obstruction was successful with a number of long-term survivors. Even younger patients maintained exercise tolerance. As of 2008, there were only 100 reported cases of apical to aortic valved conduits in the English language literature.[13-18]

The hemodynamic performance of valved conduits is well-studied. Valved conduits do not impair ventricular function, they reduce concomitant mitral valvular regurgitation by at least one grade, and they allow for 65% of the cardiac output to flow through the low resistance conduit. Interestingly, the progression of native aortic valve stenosis is arrested after placement of an apicoaortic conduit.[12, 19]

Consideration of apicoaortic conduits is appealing for a number of reasons: first, for patients with a porcelain aorta the risk of stroke from aortic cross-clamping or hypothermic circulatory arrest are minimized. Secondly, the deleterious effects of cardiopulmonary bypass and associated renal failure are avoided. Finally, transfemoral aortic valves (TAVI) are not widely available and their use is plagued by a high incidence of stroke as well as vascular access issues. The construction of apicoaortic conduits utilizes a blend of techniques found in cardiac, vascular, and thoracic surgery, and the technical difficulty of this operation has prevented its widespread acceptance; however, in a very select subset of patients, this procedure can provide survival benefits.

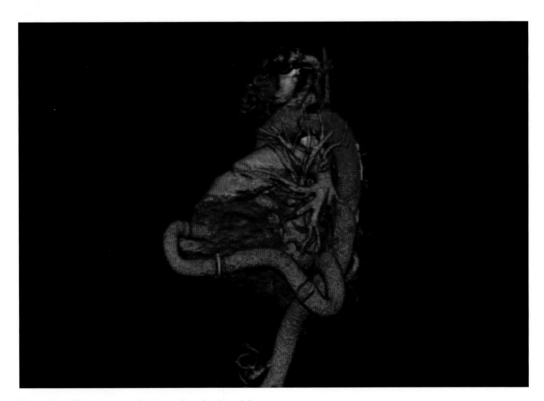

Figure 22-2 CT angiogram of apicoaortic valved conduit.

COMMENTARY

(Baron L. Hamman, Dallas, TX) Use of an apex to aorta conduit is not new. The first reports were made in children. A recent report of long term follow up of 7 cases from Texas Heart showed that properly implanted apex-to-aorta conduits can greatly benefit patients and allow the native tissue to grow or change without cicatrix or pannus or mechanical problems at the site of the aortic root.

Recent interest (financial investment) in percutaneous implanted aortic valves (TAVI) on the heels of the huge success of coronary stenting has fueled a zealous interest in the technique. Some have now even revised the definition of the "inoperable" patient. Because the STS and European data bases consistently underestimate the risk of the "high risk" aortic valve replacement patient an additional evaluation – the Frailty Index (Mike Mack, Dallas, Texas) – has been conceived and used to stratify patients for the Partners (Edwards) and CoreValve (Medtronic) trials. Percutaneous techniques have consistently shown a risk of perioperative stroke from 5% to 33% and paravalvular leaks in 12 to 30%. There is no difference in longevity in the operated vs. medically treated cohorts in the trials.

Apical to aortic valve conduits have been recently re-developed by a handful of skillful surgeons. With 1/3 of blood flowing past the untouched aortic root and 2/3 of the LV blood flow coursing through the conduit the shared load allows perfusion of the coronary arteries, likely antegrade from the aortic root to the head vessels – even during the implantation. Gammie (Maryland) and Brown (Indiana) have shown definitively that the aortic valve bypass (apical – aortic conduit) can be performed with minimal morbidity and mortality with no leaks and with no stroke. With their development of a hand held apical applicator they have been able to perform the operation without the use of cardiopulmonary bypass. There is great promise for this technique in competent hands.

REFERENCES

1. U.S. Census Bureau. 2008. U.S. Population Projections. www.census.gov/population/www.projection/2008projections.html.

2. Bouma BJ, Renee BA, VandenBrink, RB, et al. Which elderly patients with severe aortic stenosis benefit from surgical treatment? An aid to clinical decision making. *J Heart Valve Disease.* 2004; 13:374-381.

3. Asimakopoulos G, Edwards MB, Taylor KM. Aortic valve replacement in patients 80 years of age and older: Survival and cause of death based on 1100 cases. Collective results from the UK heart valve registry. *Circulation.* 1997; 96: 3403-3408.

4. Charlson E, Legedza AT., Hamel MB. Decision-making and outcomes in severe symptomatic aortic stenosis. *J Heart Valve Disease.* 2006; 15: 312-321.

5. Varadarajan P, Kapoor N, Bansal RC, et al. Survival in elderly patients with severe aortic stenosis is dramatically improved by aortic valve replacement: Results from a cohort of 277 patients aged > or + 80 years. *Eur J Cardiothoracic Surg.* 2006; 30: 722-727.

6. Melby SJ, Zieler A, Kaiser SP, et al. Aortic valve replacement in octogenarians: Risk factor for early and later mortality. *Ann Thorac Surg.* 2007; 83: 1651-1657.

7. Mortasawi A, Gehle S, Schroder T, et al. Aortic valve replacement in 80- and over 80-year-old patients. Short-term and long-term results. *Z Gerontol Geriatr.* 2000; 33: 438-446.

8. Feldman T, Leon MB. Prospects for percutaneous valve therapies. *Circulation.* 2007; 116: 2866-2877.

9. Morell VO, Duggett WM, Pezzella AT, et al. Aortic stenosis in the elderly: Results of aortic valve replacement. *J Cardiovasc Surg (Torino).* 1996; 37 (suppl2): 33-35.

10. Gammie JS, Brown JW, Brown JM, et al. Aortic valve bypass for the high-risk patient with aortic stenosis. *Ann Thorac Surg.* 2006; 81: 1605-1610.

11. Varadarajan P, Kapoor N, Ramesh C, et al. Clinical profile land natural history of 453 nonsurgically managed patients with severe aortic stenosis. *Ann Thorac Surg.* 2006; 82: 2111-215.

12. Vliek CJ, Balaras E, Li S, et al. Early and midterm hemodynamics after aortic valve bypass (apicoaortic conduit) surgery. *Ann Thorac Surg.* 2010; 90: 136-143.

13. Brown JW, Girod DA, Hurwitz RA, et al. Apicoaortic valved conduits for complex left ventricular outflow obstruction: technical considerations and current status. *Ann Thorac Surg.* 1984; 38: 162-168.

14. Gammie JS, Brown JW, Brown JM, et al. *Hemodynamic efficacy of the aortic valve bypass (apicoaortic conduit): Assessment by 2D Doppler echocardiography.* San Francisco, CA: Int Soc Min Invas Card Surg; 2006.

15. Gammie JS, Krowsoskils, Brown JM, et al. Aortic valve bypass surgery: Midterm clinical outcomes in a high-risk aortic stenosis population. *Circulation.* 2008; 118: 1460-1466.

16. Sweeney MS, Walker WE, Cooley DA, et al. Apicoaortic conduits for complex left ventricular outflow obstruction: 10-year experience. *Ann Thorac Surg.* 1986; 42: 609-611.

17. Cooley DA, Lopez RM, Absi TS. Apicoaortic conduit for left ventricular outflow tract obstruction: revisited. *Ann Thorac Surg.* 2000; 69: 1511-1514.

18. Crestanello JA, Zehr KJ, Daly RC, et al. Is there a role for the left ventricle apical-aortic conduit for acquired aortic stenosis? *J Heart Valve Dis.* 2004; 13: 57-63.

19. Caulery PJ, Otto CM. Prevention of calcified aortic valve stenosis – fact or fiction? *Ann Med.* 2009; 41: 100-108.

20. Brown JW, Gammie JS. *Off-pump aortic valve bypass using a valved apical-aortic conduit. Operative technique in thoracic and cardiovascular surgery.* Philadelphia, PA: Saunders Elsevier; 2007.

CHAPTER 23

The Future of Endovascular Aortic Therapy

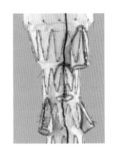

Intelligence is important,
imagination is indispensable.
– Albert Einstein

The impact of endovascular aortic therapy in the last decade has been nothing short of remarkable. Between the years 2000 and 2005, there was a 600% increase in the number of endovascular AAA repairs performed in United States hospitals.[1] Abdominal aortic aneurysm repair by EVAR has become a routine operation that is associated with a minimal mortality risk even among octogenarians. In many situations, EVAR can be performed with conscious sedation and local anesthesia alone. An even greater relative reduction in morbidity and mortality is found when comparing TEVAR to the open repair of TAAs. The advances in TEVAR therapy are more impressive when considering TEVAR is a procedure that is truly in its infancy, with the first thoracic stent graft approved by the FDA in March 2005. The relative simplicity and safety of basic EVAR have allowed these techniques to become quickly disseminated throughout the community hospital system and not remain concentrated in academic centers.

GENETIC TESTING AND SCREENING

As discussed in more detail in Chapters 1 and 7, many aneurysms have a genetic component. Aneurysms have been identified as occurring within syndromes such as Marfan, Ehlers-Danlos-IV, and Loeys-Dietz syndromes. Aneurysms which occur as part of a syndrome are linked to a specific gene mutation. Familial aneurysms are not linked to a specific syndrome, but rather these aneurysms are found clustered around first or second degree relatives within a family. Familial aneurysms have been linked to a number of different gene mutations in ACTA2, MYH11, and TGFBR2. Even in patients with random or sporadic occurring aneurysms there has been found to have an increased chance of having a duplication in chromosome 16p13.1. Currently, a family history questionnaire to assess for aneurysms in first of second degree relatives seems prudent. In the future, the ability to perform genetic testing may become simplified, accurate, and widely available. If a blood test could determine a patients genetic propensity to develop an aneurysm, that would represent the ultimate in personalized medicine.

BIOMARKERS FOR ENDOLEAKS

Matrix metalloproteinases (MMPs) are a family of more than 25 endopeptidases that are known to degrade components of the ECM. During the last decade, MMP-2 and MMP-9 have been implicated with AAA and TAA formation and rupture. Plasma levels of MMP-9 are known to increase in patients who have a known AAA that increases in size. Plasma levels of MMP-9 are reduced after patients undergo AAA repair either by open aneurysmorraphy or EVAR. MMP-9 levels can rise again, after EVAR, if an endoleak develops.[3] The implication is that in the future plasma biomarkers can be used to assess for aneurysm enlargement or potentially to detect endoleaks after EVAR. If such technology becomes available and dependable, it could reduce the expense and radiation exposure associated with computerized tomographic surveillance.

PRESSURE SENSORS

Currently all EVAR and TEVAR patients undergo some form of life-long surveillance to assess for endoleaks, graft migration, or native aneurysm sac enlargement. Currently used methods of endograft surveillance include ultrasound, computerized tomography, and magnetic resonance angiography. MRA is expensive and is not universally accepted as a means to detect endoleaks. Ultrasound is highly dependent on the skill of the technologist and CTA involves repeated contrast and radiation exposure. Wireless pressure sensors placed within the aneurysm sac at time of TEVAR and EVAR may hold promise as a noninvasive means to obtain a specific pressure measurement from the excluded aneurysm sac.

The CardioMEMS EndoSure Wireless Pressure Sensor (CardioMEMS, Inc., Atlanta, Georgia) is a series of copper coils within a silicon matrix with a pressure sensitive surface. A hand-held device works as both a transmitter and receiver. The radio frequency energy emitted by the transmitter causes the coils to vibrate and generate a resource frequency that is dependent upon the ambient pressure (sac pressure). The antenna detects the frequency of the resonated waves and a pressure reading can be generated. The CardioMEMS is currently only approved to detect endoleaks at time of graft implantation. In my opinion the intraoperative arteriogram is more than satisfactory for that purpose; however, if wireless sensors can accurately measure sac pressure years after surgery then the need for

CT scans can be reduced significantly. Patients could theoretically undergo testing of sac pressure measurements at home in much the way pacemakers are currently interrogated. Possibly the most value of wireless pressure sensors may someday lie in their use in the congestive heart failure market. A wireless pressure sensor placed in the pulmonary artery, could be quickly interrogated by the cardiologist or emergency department physician to determine a patients degree of heart failure.

MEDICAL THERAPY OF ANEURYSMS

Along with tobacco cessation, the tetracyclines may hold the most promise as a medical means to slow on stop aneurysm progression. The relationship with doxycycline as an MMP inhibitor is still not fully elucidated. What if a completely safe drug, with no side effects, were developed that could slow or prevent aneurysm growth? At what diameter of aneurysm would such a drug be given? Would such a drug be used prophylactically?

BRANCHED AND FENESTRATED ENDOGRAFTS

Branched and fenestrated grafts are not currently approved for use in the United States. Although these grafts are often discussed together, they are actually quite different. Fenestrated grafts have "holes" or ports on the side of the main body of the graft. The configuration of the ports are usually constructed as pre-ordered and custom-made for the individual patients anatomy. The ports must have an extremely accurate axial alignment with the ostia of the arterial side branches.

Branched grafts tend to have two general configurations. Some graft branched are longer and are designed to extend directly into the side branch artery. Other grafts have short branch limbs that are directed into the "general vicinity" of the arterial side branches. A second connecting covered graft is used to extend the short graft branch into the arterial side branch. The short graft limbs may be able to accommodate a wider anatomic variance that the fenestrated grafts with no branches because they do not need strict axial alignment. Thus with short side branch grafts; a few sizes may fit most. Another theoretical advantage of the short branched grafts is that they may be more tolerant of aortic movement

and angulation over time. Thus they may have a durability advantage over the nonbranched fenestrated system. Figure 23-1 is an illustration of the Cook fenestrated graft (Cook Medical Inc., Bloomington, In.). Figure 23-2 is a photo of the Cook branched graft. It is through the short branches that the renal and mesenteric arteries may be cannulated and the branches extended.

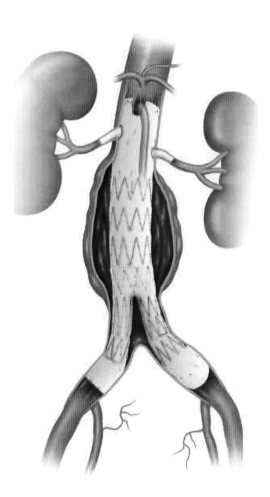

Figure 23-1 Illustration of the fenestrated graft system for thoracoabdominal aortic aneurysms. Courtesy Cook Medical Inc., Bloomington, IN.

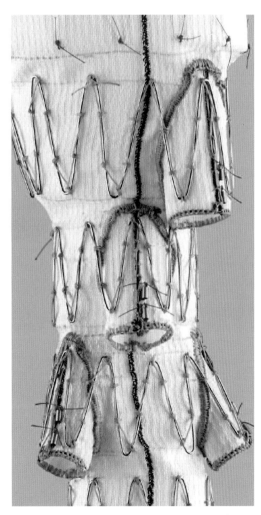

Figure 23-2 Photograph of the branched graft system for cannulation of renal and mesenteric arteries. Courtesy Cook Medical Inc., Bloomington, IN.

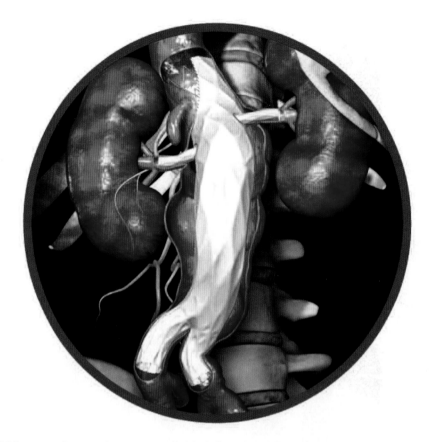

Figure 23-3 Ventana graft system. Image courtesy Endologix Corp., Irvine, CA.

VENTANA GRAFT

The Ventana graft (Endologix Corp. Irvine, Ca.) is a covered stent graft with an open or uncovered scalloped anterior portion to allow for unobstructed blood flow into the celiac and superior mesenteric arteries. Covered grafts extend into the renal arteries, figure 23-3. This graft is designed primarily to treat juxtarenal AAAs.

MEDTRONIC BRANCHED GRAFT

Another example of branched graft technology is this concept graft from Medtronic Corp. Santa Rosa, CA., figure 23-4. This graft is not in production and not available for use. This photo represents a "concept graft" to illustrate branched technology.

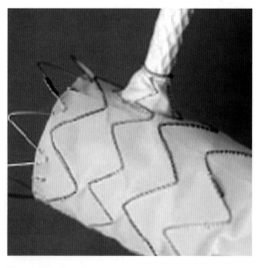

Figure 23-4 Branched "concept graft." Photograph courtesy Medtronic Inc., Santa Rosa, CA.

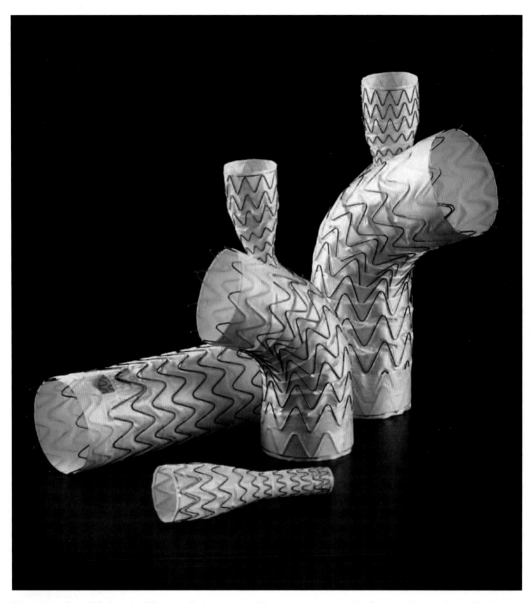

Figure 23-5 Gore TAG Branched Thoracic Endoprosthesis. Photograph courtesy W.L. Gore and Assoc., Flagstaff, AZ.

GORE BRANCHED THORACIC GRAFT

The Gore TAG Branched Thoracic Endoprosthesis (W.L Gore and Assoc. Flagstaff, AZ) is a modular stent graft system which includes both an aortic component and a single side-branch component, figure 23-5. This graft is not currently approved for use in the United States. Although intended for the side branch to be placed in the left subclavian artery, with a little imagination one could visualize the side branch placed within the innominate artery or the left carotid artery in conjunction with a debranching procedure.

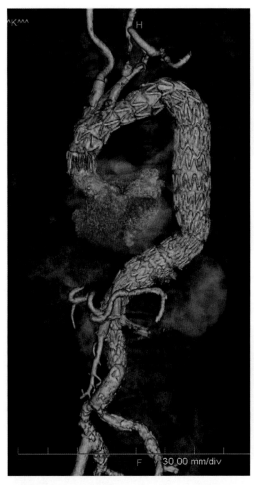

Figure 23-6 Branched Endovascular aortic arch and branched endovascular thoracoabdominal aortic repairs. Image courtesy Timothy Chuter.

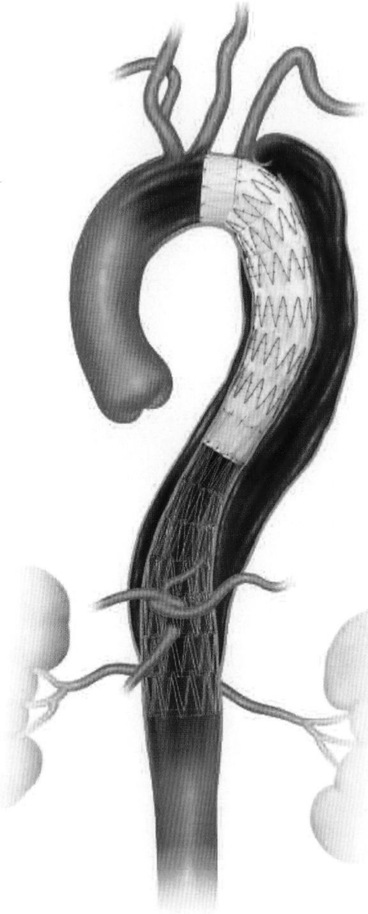

Figure 23-7 Aortic dissection system. Zenith TX2 stent graft proximally with open Z-Stents distally. Illustration courtesy Cook Medical Inc., Bloomington, IN.

BRANCHED THORACIC GRAFTS

Branched ascending and transverse arch endografts are being developed, one version involves delivering a branched ELG into the ascending aorta via the right common aortic artery. Branches for the left aortic or left subclavian artery can also be constructed. These grafts can be extended through the transverse arch and/or descending aorta. The CTA, figure 23-6, demonstrates such a graft placed in the ascending aorta of a patient who three years prior had a complete endovascular repair of the thoracoabdominal aorta with a branched endograft.

TEVAR FOR AORTIC DISSECTION

Endografting for aortic dissection is not approved in the United States, although it is commonly performed at select centers. Chapters 14 and 15 outline some basic principles of aortic dissection and endovascular dissection repair. Figure 23-7 is the Cook Dissection System. The Cook system uses a Zenith TX2 component proximally and bare metal Z-stents as the distal component. The open Z-stents permit blood flow into the aortic side branches and also gradually appose the true and false lumens.

E-VITA GRAFT

The E-vita graft (JOTEC, Hechingen, Germany) consists of a polyester covered stent graft on one end and an unstented polyester graft on the other end, figure 23-8. the stented portion can be placed into the true lumen of an aortic dissection in an antegrade fashion under direct vision. The stent graft could also be placed over a guidewire previously delivered retrograde with IVUS guidance to ensure true lumen placement. The unstented proximal portion of the polyester graft can accept the head vessels sutured together or an island patch. Alternatively, a bifurcated or trifurcated graft can be sutured to the great vessels individually and then sutured to the proximal portion of the E-vita graft. Because the distal stent-containing portion of the graft is "fixed" within the descending thoracic aorta, as opposed to free-floating, the technique is known as the "frozen elephant trunk".

NITINOL VERSUS STAINLESS STEEL

Endografts with a stainless steel skeleton could be expected to have a durability advantage over nitinol-based stent grafts. Stainless steel can exist within the human body and essentially not degrade. Nitinol can deteriorate over 25 to 30 years. However, the "all cause mortality" related to co-morbidities precludes most patients from living greater than 30 years after aneurysm repair. Nitinol has the advantage of being more compressible and thus nitinol devices can have a "low profile" and potentially be delivered through smaller sheaths. Obviously nitinol-based stent systems would appeal to some manufacturers as lower profile systems would allow EVAR to become fully percutaneous and theoretically make EVAR more accessible to nonsurgical specialties.

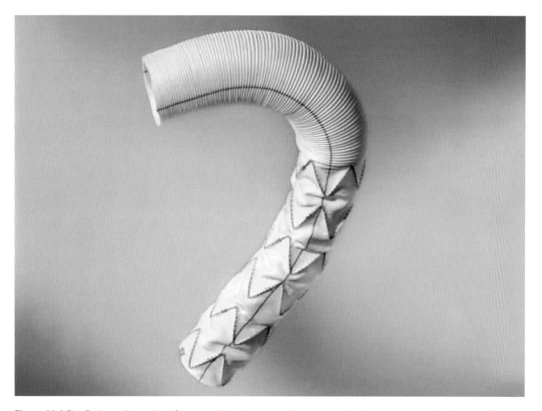

Figure 23-8 The E-vita graft consists of a covered stent on one end an unstented polyester tube on the other end. The covered stent can be placed into the proximal descending thoracic aorta to construct the "frozen elephant trunk".

MULTILAYER FLOW MODULATOR

What may be the most successful next generation stent graft may not have a "fabric" or "covered" coating. This device is technically not a stent but a multilayer flow modulator (Cardiatis, Isnes, Belgium). This is a 3-dimensional structure composed of three layers of chromium alloy filaments that are interwoven to each other, figure 23-9. When placed within an artery containing an aneurysm, they decrease the flow vortex within the aneurysm sac. Ninety percent of the blood flow becomes laminar within the multilayer stent and only 10% of the blood flow reaches the aneurysm sac.

When blood flows out of the first layer of the multilayer stent its pressure decreases by delta P1. When blood flows out of the second layer the pressure decreases by delta P2. The pressure decreases by delta P3 as the blood leaves the third layer of the stent. The reduced flow and pressure within the sac results in thrombosis of the aneurysm sac. Interestingly, arterial side branches that may be covered by the device are able to maintain their flow and remain patent. Multilayer flow modulators are manufactured in diameters of 2 mm to 40 mm and have been used to treat popliteal, cerebral, and renal aneurysms.[4-6] One report describes the use of a multilayer flow modulator in a residual type B aortic dissection. In that case the false lumen thrombosed while maintaining patency of the visceral side branch arteries.[7]

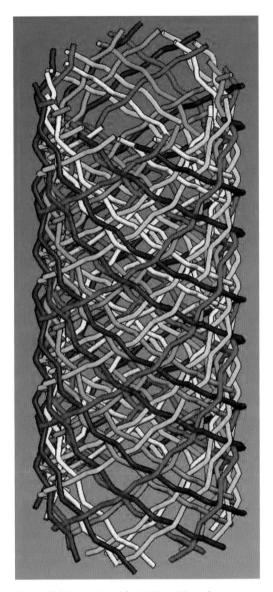

Figure 23-9 Illustration of Cardiatis multilayer flow modulator.[4]

COMMENTARY

(Edward B. Diethrich, Phoenix, AZ) The Multilayer Flow Modulator truly represents a disruptive technology. Dr. Mitchell clearly explains the physics of flow upon which this modulator concept is based. My personal experience with the device in the preclinical laboratory studies and a handful of human applications as well as knowledge of the current worldwide clinical cases, leads me to believe the concept, when tested in well controlled trials, will prove a valuable tool in our vascular practices.

REFERENCES

1. Nowygrod R, Egorova N, Greco G, et al. Trends, complications, and mortality in peripheral vascular surgery. *J Vasc Surg.* 2006; Feb 43 (2): 205-216.

2. Sangiorgi G, D'Averio R, Maureiello A, et al. Plasma levels of metalloproteinases -3 and -9 as markers of successful abdominal aortic aneurysm exclusion after endovascular graft treatment. *Circulation.* 2001; 104 (12 Suppl. 1): 1288-1295.

3. Lorelli DR, Jean-Claude JM, Fox CJ, et al. Response of plasma matrix metalloproteinase -9 to conventional abdominal aortic aneurysm repair or endovascular exclusion: Implication for endoleak. *J Vasc Surg.* 2002; 35: 916.

4. Wailliez C and Coussement G. CFD study of multilayer stent haemodynamics effects in abdominal aortic aneurysms. *NCTAM;* 2006.

5. Henry M, Polydorou A, Frid N, et al. Treatment of renal artery aneurysms with the multilayer stent. *J Endovasc Ther.* 2008; 15: 231-236.

6. Polydorou A, Henry M, Bellenis I, et al. Endovascular treatment of arterial aneurysms with side branch: A simple method. Myth or reality. *Hospital Chronicles.* 5; 2: 88-94.

7. Chocron S, Vaislic C, Kaili D, Bonneville JF. Multilayer stents in the treatment of thoracoabdominal residual type B dissection. *Interact Cardiovasc Thorac Surg.* 2011; 12: 1057-1059.

About the Author

Robert Owen Mitchell was born in Frankfort, Kentucky. He graduated with a bachelor's degree from Centre College in Danville, Kentucky. He received his master's degree in biochemistry and his doctoral degree in medicine at the University of Louisville in Louisville, Kentucky. Dr. Mitchell completed his residency in general surgery and cardiothoracic surgery at the University of Louisville. Currently, Dr. Mitchell resides in Lexington, Kentucky with his wife and two daughters. He has been in the private practice of cardiothoracic and vascular surgery for 17 years.